I am diabetic. This program has enabled me to reduce my daily insulin by 3 units per day and has eliminated my need for insulin coverage during the day. I am waking with fasting glucoses of 95 or less. This all happened in two weeks on this program. Every diabetic should take a serious look at this program, it is life saving!

I am sleeping better, have lost 5 lbs and my pants now feel comfortable on me. My shoulder was hurting before I started the class, it was difficult for me to lift my arm over my head to take my shirts on and off and now I have no pain at all.

This is the first time EVER in my life that I have found an eating plan that I am so totally happy with that I see myself easily sustaining this plan indefinitely.

It has been years since I have felt as good as I do now. Just having the knowledge of knowing why to eat what I eat and when to eat is a really big deal for me. For ages I would tell myself that if only I could get to around 175, I would feel great. Now I weigh 155 and it just feels right. Mainly though, I just love the food, the routine, the diet.

I have rheumatoid arthritis and went to my doctor yesterday. He was pleased with my 12 pound weight loss and decrease in hand pain. He is lowering my pred from 5 mg/day to 4 mg/day and then down to 3! Yeah! My blood pressure has also shown improvement.

Since taking your class, I have steadily lost 25 pounds over the year— while eating healthy and delicious food. It has been wonderful to feel satisfied and have a healthy tummy (no acid reflux) while going down 3 sizes nearly effortlessly.

We are doing great here. I've introduced the TQI Diet to my adult daughters. My oldest has asthma that has gotten better. What a transformative experience. We will never look at food the same way again. We continue to watch our weight go down and our clothes FALL DOWN! We've also had record low blood pressure readings in doctor's office: 110/68. It's all quite amazing.

What we got from the TQI Diet that is so much more important than the weight loss, is our new relationship, perspective and appreciation for food.

One of the best things I've noticed so far about the diet is a feeling of lightness in my stomach. I think I spend a lot of time feeling heavy and bloated during my normal life so this is refreshing.

I have been losing weight even though I am eating a lot. I don't feel deprived—in fact, I am enjoying food more than ever!

The most remarkable thing for me is that as someone who has struggled with my weight most of my adult life, all the little voices in my head are quieting down: "Am I eating too much?" "Am I eating too little?" "Should I be eating now?" "Should I not be eating now?" I am no longer worried about what I am eating. The balance in my nourishment has created a balance in my thinking about food and every meal is great.

This diet is sustainable unlike other diets I have tried and I feel like I can make solid life style changes with it.

Though not perfectly, I have followed your program quite well— and with amazing results. thought it would be nice to achieve my college graduation weight. I am at that weight. Ten years ago my cholesterol had ballooned up to 280. At a recent physical after having followed your program my cholesterol had dropped to 154.

I took the course to find a solution to my PCOS symptoms. I had been dealing with fertility issues as well as weight gain for about 5 years. After 3 months on the TQI diet, my cycles regulated and I got pregnant. I am now 20 weeks along! Baby is growing right on track, and my midwife is impressed!

THE ABASCAL WAY
To Quiet Inflammation

Kathy Abascal

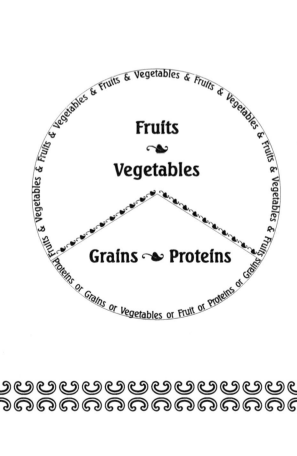

Publisher: Tigana Press, P.O. Box 1528, Vashon, WA 98070.
Printed in the United States of America.
First Edition

ISBN: 9780978858605
LCCN: 2010938055

Front cover photograph:
A Path Through Darkness Often Leads to a Brighter Future
© ① ◎ by Brian J Buck

Back cover photograph:
Archway
© ① by IrishFireside

NOTE: This book contains the opinions and ideas of its author. It is intended to provide informative material on the subject covered, and is sold with the understanding that the author and publisher are not rendering professional services in the book. If the reader requires personal assistance or advice, an appropriate professional should be consulted. A competent health care professional should always be consulted before any dietary changes are made. The author and publisher specifically disclaim any responsibility for any liability, loss, or risk, personal or otherwise, which is incurred as a consequence directly or indirectly, of the use and application of any of the contents of this book.

❧ *Dedication* ❧

First and foremost, I want to thank my good friend Manuel Abascal for helping to bring this book to fruition. He patiently worked up many edits and made many valuable suggestions on how to improve the book. Similarly, my girlfriend Joanne Berg, my mother, Jeanne Louise Shull, and my sister Holly Shull Vogel took the time to read the book over and over again for content, spelling, and grammar. They made many suggestions that improved the flow and look of the book. They kept me going when it seemed the book never would get finished. Chuck Bowden also took the time to read the manuscript and David Hinchman of Vashon Print & Design helped me over some of the technical bumps in the road to publication.

Recently, Rex Morris came bounding in with a burst of positive energy that helped carry the book to completion. Finally, I owe great thanks to my friends and students who have encouraged me to publish my book and who helped refine the content by asking interesting questions and sharing their stories and thoughts with me.

TABLE OF CONTENTS

PART ONE: INTRODUCTION

PART TWO: THE ELIMINATION PHASE

PART THREE: THE TESTING PHASE

PART FOUR: A PATH FOR LIFE

PART FIVE: APPENDICES

PART ONE
Introduction

THE ABASCAL WAY
Introduction

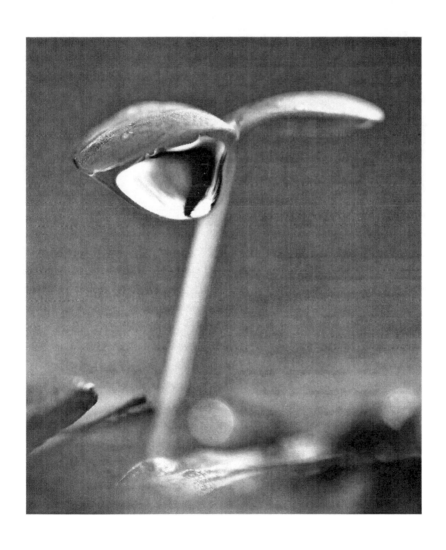

The most amazing aspect of the Abascal Way To Quiet Inflammation (the TQI Diet) is how quickly it works. We are told that our food choices will determine whether we end up with cancer or diabetes in our golden years. I certainly had known that for years and years and years. Nonetheless, on any given evening a plateful of ravioli in gorgonzola sauce, some bread to dip in the sauce, a couple of glasses of red wine, and a dessert spoke more loudly to me than what might or might not happen at some point in the future. Like Scarlett O'Hara (but with a substantially wider and ever-growing waist) I'd tell myself "I can't think about that right now. If I do, I'll go crazy. I'll think about that tomorrow."

Unfortunately, that tomorrow never really arrived because the eating choices I thought I should make were boring and any short term benefits those boring choices might bring were way too slow in coming. I would watch my calories and avoid sweets, but my weight loss was excruciatingly slow. Soon enough, I'd slip and return to my slow-but-steady weight gain pattern. Health was important to me but it was not a big motivator because frankly I thought my health was fine. I actually thought my diet was pretty good as well. I did not know that my blood pressure was creeping up alongside my weight. I had no idea that my stiff ankles and my achy frozen shoulders meant that inflammation was smoldering in my body. If I thought at all about the aches that interfered with my sleep and were starting to limit my life, I simply wrote them off as an inevitable part of aging.

But things changed when I realized that not only was I aging but my body was beginning to fall apart.[1] I was finally motivated to try to use my diet to improve my health. I knew that if I was diligent, I could reduce my blood pressure and my weight. My

---

[1] See "Author's Story" in Appendix C for more details.

research told me that diet could quiet the inflammation that was making my body ache. But, in truth, I was a skeptic. I really did not expect to make much progress on any front. Fortunately, the TQI Diet worked quickly. I began to see and feel benefits before my inner skeptic had a chance to convince me to give up.

On the TQI Diet, I began sleeping better immediately. Within days, my ankles lost their "morning stiffness" and I no longer hobbled to the kitchen to put on my morning coffee. All good, but truth be told, it was my weight loss that amazed me. I was sick of the middle-aged "thickness" that had taken over my body. Seeing the scale drop even though I was eating (gasp) cashew butter and avocados thrilled me no end. These immediate successes made me willing to continue on the diet.

Of course it helps that the TQI diet is not a boring diet. You simply try an anti-inflammatory diet for a brief period—five weeks to be exact. For five weeks, you take a break from eating the way you usually eat. You also take a break from counting calories and measuring portions, even if you have a substantial weight issue. Your only concern for these five weeks is whether a food is inflammatory or not.

We focus our efforts on reducing inflammation because medical research now shows that chronic inflammation is the engine that drives most problems of middle and old age.[2] It fuels our weight problems and many of us live with chronic pain as a result of systemic inflammation. Inflammation is a smoldering fire in our bodies. We need to stop its heat from damaging our body. At the same time, our immune system must remain able to use inflammation to fight off viruses, bacteria, and other acute diseases. We need to quiet unnecessary chronic inflammation without suppressing our immune system. The TQI diet achieves this goal quickly and elegantly.

The human body is miraculous: Given the right nutritional "tools" it immediately moves toward health. As we get healthier, everything improves. Cholesterol levels move toward normal

---

[2]   Unfortunately, these days our children usually eat poorly and experience health and weight issues that used to only afflict adults.

because healthy people have normal cholesterol levels. Blood sugar levels return to normal because healthy people are not diabetic. Blood pressure moves toward normal because healthy people are not hypertensive. And, as we get healthier, our weight moves toward normal. A healthy person is neither under- nor overweight. A healthy person is normal weight.

The reasons *why* the TQI diet works are set out in detail in the chapters that follow because knowledge is essential to your success. You need to know why your food choices matter. And when I say, "know," I mean a knowing seated deep in your bones. This type of knowing occurs when experience marries book knowledge. As you eliminate and reintroduce foods, you feel how they affect you. At the same time you learn why those foods affect you the way they do. Then later, when temptation rears its head—and it will—you will not be pulled off course. As a wise person once said: "There are neither rewards nor punishments in life, there are simply consequences." If you know the consequences of your food choices, you will make intelligent choices more often than not.

Eating this way changed my life and, as a teacher, I have again and again seen the TQI diet quickly change how my students feel and look. I sincerely hope you take the plunge and give the TQI Diet your all for five weeks. If you do, it will transform your life. At the end of five weeks, you will no longer see this as a "diet." Instead, you will choose to eat the Abascal Way because it makes you look and feel well. You simply will not want to eat any other way.

CHAPTER ONE
Intra-Abdominal Fat

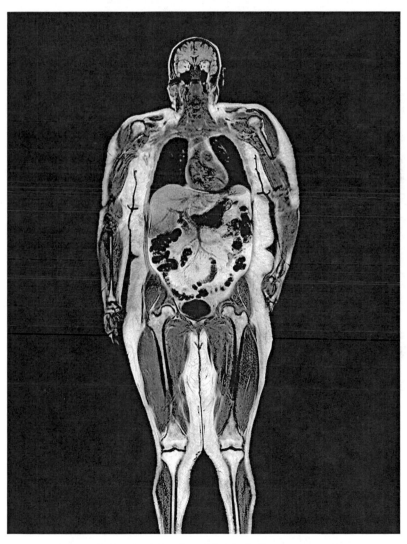

Intra-abdominal fat is a highly inflammatory fat
that even a thin person may carry.

Our culture loves the slender figure, and most of us dream of being trim and slim. Nonetheless, most of us are not slender. In fact, more than a third of Americans are obese and another third are overweight.[1] Shedding those extra pounds is important because those extra pounds put the overweight at high risk for chronic diseases, ranging from cancer to heart attacks to stroke. Statistics tell us that a waist wider than 36 inches (for a woman) or 40 inches (for a man) is a health hazard because an oversized waist means that its owner carries too much intra-abdominal fat.

Intra-abdominal fat is different than the subcutaneous fat that collects under the surface of our skin, fat that we can pinch or jiggle on our upper arms or thighs. Intra-abdominal fat is an internal fat that wraps itself around, and infiltrates our vital organs. We cannot see the fat wrapped around our heart, our liver, or our kidneys—but that fat has a dramatic, negative effect on our health because it is very inflammatory. During check-ups, our doctors remind us that we need to lose a little weight to avoid chronic disease that will make our life miserable. In response, we go on a weight-loss diet that dramatically reduces our daily calorie intake. Some of us lose weight this way but many of us do not. Of those who do, few are able to maintain their weight loss.

Intra-abdominal fat is also a problem for the underweight. Underweight people are often as inflamed as their overweight counterparts but, because only a few percent of the population are underweight, they do not receive much attention or advice despite the health problems they face. They are usually advised simply to eat more. To gain weight many turn to cakes, cookies, ice cream, smoothies, and other high-calorie foods to gain weight. Some gain weight, but many do not.

---

[1] These numbers are changing rapidly. By 2015, 75% of Americans will be overweight and at least 40% will be obese.

Less than a third of the U.S. population is normal weight. They are proud of their slender bodies and feel healthy. In fact, they are often a bit self-righteous, and frown on the lack of willpower and self-indulgence of the not-so-slender. But take note of this important news: A full 60 percent of these lovely, normal-weight individuals are now classified as obese. Yes, as obese. A new term has been coined for them. They are the *normal-weight obese*. Normal-weight obese individuals have too much intra-abdominal fat and are significantly inflamed. They too are at high risk for all chronic ailments (ranging from cancer to heart attacks).

	1. Normal-Weight	2. NWO	3. Overweight
Cytokines (pg/ml)			
TNF-alpha	20	43	56
IL-6	6	11	14
IL-1 alpha	15	27	30
IL-1 beta	5	15	19
Body Fat (%)			
Percent Body Fat	23%	35%	43%

Look at the numbers in the table above. In column one, we see a *healthy* woman's data. She is the right weight for her height. Her inflammatory cytokines are in the normal range. She carries an appropriate percentage fat on her body. Compare that with the data on an *unhealthy*, slender woman—the normal-weight obese woman in column two. She is the right weight for her height but her inflammatory cytokines are double, or triple, what they should be. She is inflamed. She also carries too much body fat for her weight. Finally, compare the normal-weight obese woman with the overweight woman in column three. This woman weighs too much. Her inflammatory cytokine levels are yet higher but they are not double or triple those of the normal-weight obese woman. The overweight woman carries more body fat. She is less healthy than the normal-weight obese woman but statistically both are unhealthy and at high—and almost equal—risk for chronic ailments because both women are inflamed.

Presently, out of about 300 million Americans, 100 million are obese, 100 million are overweight, 3 million are underweight, and 60 million are "normal-weight obese." Out of 300 million people less than 40 million are actually normal weight *and* healthy. What is going on? Simply put, our approach to weight and weight loss is wrong.

When we want to lose weight, we go on a diet. There are a myriad of diet plans to pick from. Each plan has its own twist but they all basically provide ways to cut calories. Little attention is paid to what or when we eat; the emphasis is on burning calories. Most often we buy into a weight-loss program that allows us to continue eating our favorite foods. We simply eat less: A woman who burns around 1,800 calories a day typically goes on a 1,200-calories-a-day diet. In a week she will burn at least 3,500 calories more than she ate, and will lose about a pound. She mistakenly assumes she will lose a pound of fat in the process. Unfortunately, it is easier biochemically to get calories from protein than from fat. So the dieter instead depletes protein when she overly restricts calories. She ends up a normal-weight obese person with a higher amount of body fat because her diet ate up muscle tissue as well as fat.

Then, because she continues to eat inflammatory foods and not enough anti-inflammatory foods, she remains inflamed. When she reaches her goal weight, she will join the ranks of the normal-weight obese. Most likely, she will soon tire of minding her portion sizes and counting calories. She will begin to eat more of her favorite foods, and she will gain weight. The weight she puts on will be fat. Inflammation will increase, and she will soon rejoin the ranks of the inflamed, overweight in column three.

The TQI Diet has an entirely different focus and achieves very different results. We do not eat fewer calories than we need. We do not limit portion sizes; we eat until we are full. Instead of tracking how much we eat, we remove as many inflammatory foods and chemicals as we can from our diet. We replace those foods with as many anti-inflammatory foods as we can. As the burden of inflammatory foods is removed, the body begins to function better. As we regularly provide an abundance of anti-inflammatory foods, our health improves. As our health improves, our metabolism improves, we sleep better, our aches and pains recede, and, our weight moves toward normal. For most of us, that means that our weight drops. For a few, weight will increase. For those who are normal weight, weight will not change but inflammation will be quieted. Weight problems take care of themselves because they are simply a symptom of an underlying problem—inflammation.

As you learn to provide your body with the nutrients it needs—and, of equal importance, eliminate the burden of inflammatory compounds beyond the body's ability to function—intra-abdominal fat begins to melt away. As it melts away, your immune system calms down, and inflammation is quieted. You become healthy. You achieve a healthy weight. You feel and look better.

Intra-abdominal fat, the true villain, can only be addressed through an anti-inflammatory life style. You cannot melt away this fat by simply reducing your calorie intake and losing weight. You instead must eat to quiet inflammation, and that is what you will do on the TQI diet.

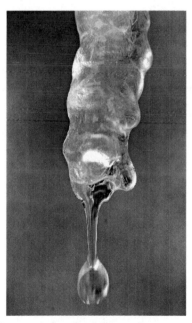

Intra-abdominal fat melts away
when we choose to eat nutrient-rich food.

CHAPTER TWO

Inflammation

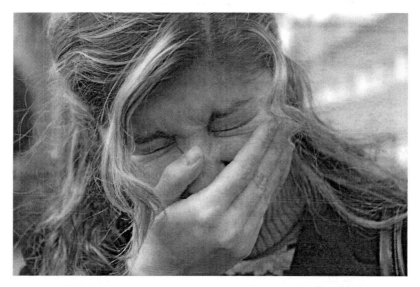

The common cold is an example of a necessary
but slightly excessive acute inflammatory response.

Inflammation is a natural part of an immune response. An acute inflammatory response protects the body from invasion and is inherently good but is sometimes too strong or slightly misdirected.[1] In contrast, chronic inflammation is as a rule neither necessary nor desirable. Chronic inflammation increases our intra-abdominal fat, makes us feel poorly, and heightens the likelihood that we will develop diabetes, high blood pressure, and other health problems. Chronic inflammation is rampant in the United States and needs to be reduced.

The TQI diet works to quiet chronic inflammation, and is based on three principles: Eat the right foods, eat the right proportions of those foods, and eat at the right time. Basically, when we give our body the right foods in the right balance, our body functions better, and we immediately reduce inflammation. As inflammation quiets, we experience less pain, better sleep, more energy during the day, and we feel better overall. So let us begin our journey by looking at inflammation: What exactly is it?

Our immune system, working constantly to defend our health, uses a complicated feedback system to trigger or quiet inflammation as needed. The immune system consists of billions of cells that use chemicals called cytokines as their messengers. Some cytokines increase inflammation while others quiet it. Whether we are inflamed depends on the complex balance of our cytokines at any given moment.

THREE ACUTE INFLAMMATORY RESPONSES

An acute inflammatory response is set in motion when microbes move into our body, such as when we suffer a wound, catch a cold, or come down with the flu.

---

[1] *Acute* is a word used to describe an injury or illness that comes and goes (as opposed to *chronic*, which is persistent).

1. OUR IMMUNE RESPONSE TO A WOUND

Wounds break the skin and open the body up to the outside world. Our skin surface is covered with bacteria that immediately take advantage of the opening and invade. We keep immune cells positioned throughout the body to detect and respond to such bacterial invasions. The resident immune cells immediately begin to engulf and kill the invading bacteria but more immune cells are needed to fight off the stream of invading bacteria. The resident immune cells therefore begin secreting cytokines that diffuse into the blood stream and travel throughout the body. These cytokines attract other immune cells to the wound site to help fight off the invaders.

Immune cells are relatively large and must push their way out of the blood vessels and between the cells of the tissue to reach the wound site. The inflammatory cytokines "loosen up the tissue" a bit for these cells, but much of the work is done mechanically by the immune cells squeezing their way through the tissue. This disrupts the tissue, causing some of the swelling, redness, and pain of the wound. Once at the wound site, immune cells begin killing bacteria. As the number of bacteria dwindle, the immune cells stop producing inflammatory cytokines because additional immune cells are not needed. Once the bacteria are vanquished, the surplus immune cells leave. The wound scabs over, and the redness, the swelling and the pain disappear. Things return to normal. This is a perfect acute immune response with just enough of an inflammatory response to protect and heal the body. Although the inflammatory response momentarily adds to the discomfort of the wound, the discomfort is outweighed by the benefit of preventing bacteria from taking over the body.

2. OUR RESPONSE TO THE COMMON COLD

The common cold is caused by viruses that replicate in the upper respiratory passages. They typically cause little damage to that tissue but we cannot have viral factories set up in our bodies eating up our resources, even if they cause little collateral damage. When resident immune cells detect the cold virus, they secrete inflammatory cytokines to attract more immune cells to help fight the rapidly replicating virus. The immune cells, as in the wound described above, must muscle their way through the tissue, causing some redness, swelling, and discomfort. The inflammatory cytokines help loosen up the tissue but at the same time cause the symptoms of the common cold. The congestion, runny nose and eyes, and slight fatigue that come with a cold are actually the side effects of inflammatory cytokines circulating through the body. Our cold symptoms are not directly caused by the cold virus. Once the immune system defeats the cold virus, production of inflammatory cytokines stops, and the cold symptoms dissipate.

This is a necessary but imperfect acute inflammatory response. Ideally, we would fight off the cold virus without creating uncomfortable cold symptoms. We would feel better if our inflammatory immune response were just a touch gentler. Some plant compounds may actually moderate our reaction to the cold virus: Echinacea (*Echinacea angustifolia*)[2] is an herb often used to fight colds, and is said to work by stimulating our immune response to the cold virus. Studies now indicate that, in cold-infected cells, echinacea instead reduces the production of inflammatory cytokines. It quiets some of the excessive aspects of the inflammatory response without suppressing the immune system's ability to fight the virus. In the process, it may quiet annoying cold symptoms.

3. OUR RESPONSE TO INFLUENZA

The flu virus is a difficult virus that poses a serious threat because it penetrates deeply into the respiratory tract and causes significant damage to that tissue. We need a strong immune response to fight the flu and prevent secondary problems, such as pneumonia, from developing. And our immune system responds vigorously to the flu virus, producing massive amounts of inflammatory cytokines that bring large numbers of immune cells to the respiratory tract. Once again, as in the cold, it is these cytokines that cause our flu symptoms. The severe headache,

---

[2] Plants have at least two names: A common name and a Latin name. In this book, the Latin name follows in parentheses after the plant's common name.

extreme fatigue, joint and muscle aches, and the high fever are all side effects of the inflammatory cytokines released in response to the virus; these symptoms are not directly caused by the flu virus itself.

In fact, in pandemic flu, death results when the immune system overreacts to a new strain of the flu. When confronted with a pandemic strain (such as the flu of 1918, bird flu, or difficult cases of swine flu), the immune system occasionally cycles out of control, and produces so many inflammatory cytokines that the body is destroyed in the process. This is often referred to as a cytokine storm. Our inflammatory immune response is necessary to prevent the flu virus from destroying our respiratory tissue but our inflammatory response causes substantial discomfort and sometimes death. It is a response that we might wish to quiet somewhat but one we should not suppress.

THREE CHRONIC INFLAMMATORY RESPONSES

Our immune system monitors everything that goes on in the body, and it will try to fix anything that is not working properly. It fights viruses, bacteria, protozoa, and other parasites that threaten us but our immune system also reacts to problems ranging from joint damage to diabetes and migraines to emotional stress. The immune system response always includes inflammation—thus every disease condition generates some inflammation.

Unfortunately, the immune system is not able to repair or correct the chronic problems that trouble us. Unlike an acute response to a wound, a cold, or the flu, our inflammatory response cannot solve such problems. Instead, chronic problems persist, and our inflammatory response to them persists, day after day, year after year. This exposes us to ongoing, nonproductive inflammation. Fortunately, we can quiet this type of nonproductive inflammation with diet. Three examples of chronic inflammatory responses—osteoarthritis, atherosclerosis, and food sensitivities—follow.

1. OSTEOARTHRITIS

If we damage cartilage in a joint, we set the stage for osteoarthritis. Immune cells will immediately discover the damage and try to fix it. When they are unsuccessful, they secrete inflammatory cytokines to call in yet more immune cells to help solve the problem. Much of the redness, swelling, and pain around the joint are caused by these immune cells moving toward the site of the torn cartilage. This inflammatory response is chronic—it continues day after day—for as long as the damaged cartilage remains in the body, but it never solves the problem. To make matters worse, the immune cells secrete an enzyme that further degrades the cartilage.

This is an example of a chronic, destructive inflammatory response that can be quieted with food. As diet quiets the chronic inflammatory response, it quiets much of the pain and discomfort of osteoarthritis. It also reduces some of the additional long-term damage that would otherwise be caused by enzymes secreted by the immune cells.

2. ATHEROSCLEROSIS

Our cardiovascular system's goal is to keep our blood flowing smoothly through the body. The walls of healthy blood vessels are smooth and carry a slight negative charge. The red blood cells also carry a negative charge and are slightly repelled by the negatively charged vessel walls. There is not too much sticky fat in the bloodstream. This allows the blood to bounce along without sticking and forming clots.

Sometimes a blood vessel wall is damaged. The body responds by covering the lesion with a layer of fat. This is called a fatty streak and is the beginning of atherosclerosis. Immune cells soon discover the fat stuck to the vessel wall and begin to remove it. As they absorb the fat, the body puts a new layer of fat down. As the resident immune cells fill up with fat, they begin secreting inflammatory cytokines to attract more immune cells to the site. These cells help consume the fat, and transform themselves into fat-filled foam cells that grow in size, aggregate, and form plaque. The plaque narrows the blood vessel, impairing blood flow in that part of the body. If the plaque becomes large and fibrous enough, it may break free and travel through the body as a clot. If that clot lodges in the heart, it will cause a heart attack. If it lodges in the brain, it causes a stroke.

Once again, this inflammatory response aggravates an existing problem. It is another example of a non-productive, chronic inflammatory response that we can quiet with food.

3. FOOD SENSITIVITIES

All cells—whether human, animal, plant, bacterial, viral, or fungal—have unique sugars and proteins on their surfaces. Our immune system distinguishes our own cells from foreign (or "not-self") cells based on the unique structures of these sugars and proteins. To maintain this system—which allows the immune system to fight off foreign cells but not attack its own—we do not absorb whole proteins or whole complex sugars from our diet. Instead, when we eat, we break down proteins and complex sugars into their very basic building blocks before we absorb them. We then use those building blocks to make our own unique sugars and proteins.

Our intestinal cells line up tightly next to each other to prevent larger, undigested food molecules and bacteria from entering the body. The immune system patrols the intestinal tract carefully to fight off any foreign entities that may make it through that barrier. It distinguishes between what belongs in the body (basic building blocks, our own cells, and our own proteins) and what does not (bacteria, viruses, protozoa) by the unique protein structures on their surfaces.

Problems can arise if our digestion is off-kilter and we do not fully break down our food. If our intestinal lining is inflamed and porous (because we have digestive ailments or are eating foods that disagree with us) it may allow whole foreign proteins to get through the intestinal barrier. Whole foreign proteins are a signal to the immune system that the body is being invaded. In response, the immune system mounts a strong inflammatory response and attracts large numbers of immune cells to the digestive tract to halt the invasion. The immune system also creates permanent antibody memory of the food protein, leading to a "true" food allergy. After that, each time the person eats that food or a food containing that protein, a quick and stronger response will be mounted that eventually can build to anaphylactic shock. The person has a food allergy and must carefully avoid that food.

Sometimes only parts of proteins slip into the body. This does not cause a strong allergic reaction but it does trigger an inflammatory response. The immune system is troubled because a "foreigner" has invaded the body. It is aware that other similar "foreigners" are in the intestines and may be preparing to invade the body. In response, the immune system secretes cytokines to make sure enough immune cells are present should an invasion take place. It does not, however, form a permanent antibody memory against the food. Instead of an escalating allergic response, the person simply experiences inflammation every time they eat that particular food. They have a food sensitivity.

Food sensitivities trigger inflammation and the release of the same cytokines a cold or the flu does, albeit in different amounts. Depending on the resulting specific balance of inflammatory cytokines in the individual, food sensitivities may manifest as congestion, headaches, joint aches, or any number of other symptoms. This is another nonproductive inflammatory response—the food is not preparing to invade the body—and it is a chronic inflammatory response that can be controlled with diet.

QUIETING CHRONIC INFLAMMATION

Chronic inflammation is expressed in many different ways. A child with asthma suffers from chronic inflammation. A woman with migraines and hot flashes suffers from chronic inflammation, as does an overweight man with Type II diabetes. An overworked, sleep-deprived adult has chronic inflammation. Any ongoing problem that cannot be "fixed" by an inflammatory immune response results in a degree of chronic inflammation that does not serve us well, it harms us. Fortunately, the right food choices can quiet chronic inflammation without suppressing our immune system. If we eat properly, we can feel better and be healthy, without compromising our body's ability to mend wounds and fend off infections and illnesses. In fact, by quieting inflammation, we are better able to activate and tolerate an acute inflammatory response when needed.

Our acute immune response improves because a body provided with the right balance of nutritional compounds functions optimally. A healthy body has a healthy cytokine balance. When a problem arises and the immune system produces inflammatory cytokines, its response will only result in mild symptoms. In contrast, a person eating inflammatory foods, without needed nutrients, will always have higher levels of inflammatory cytokines— resulting in discomfort on a regular basis. Then, when a problem arises that triggers a flood of inflammatory cytokines, the levels of inflammatory cytokines end up at much higher levels than in a healthier person. These high levels of inflammatory cytokines cause them to suffer greater discomfort and increase the likelihood that their body will begin to malfunction.

The ultimate goal of the TQI diet is to improve how you feel and function. In the chapters that follow, you will learn how your food choices determine how inflamed you are. This knowledge, combined with the benefits you experience while following the TQI diet, are important because we need to both understand and experience the potential benefits before we will actually make lasting changes to our eating habits.

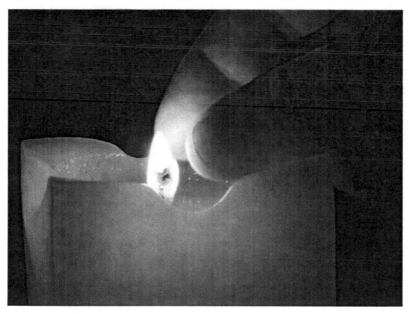

The right food choices extinguish inflammation.

PART TWO
The Elimination Phase

CHAPTER THREE

Summary of Rules
for the
3-Week Elimination Phase

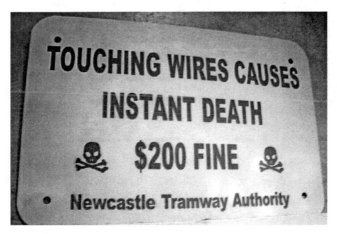

Every food choice we make has a consequence...
sometimes for the good, sometimes not.

SEVEN SIMPLE RULES GOVERN YOUR MEALS

RULE NO. ONE:

Eat only foods on the approved food lists and eat them in the proportions indicated on those lists.

RULE NO. TWO:

Eat breakfast, lunch, dinner, and two snacks each day.

RULE NO. THREE:

Eat your breakfast as soon as possible after rising. The remainder of your meals and snacks may be scheduled throughout the day to fit your needs.

RULE NO. FOUR:

Eat only at meals and snacks. In between meals and snacks, do not eat or drink anything, including "whiteners" in your beverages, mints, chewable vitamins, or gum.

RULE NO. FIVE:

Between meals and snacks you may drink water, mineral water (unsweetened, without natural or artificial flavors), and un-doctored coffee, tea, or herbal tea. You may add a squeeze of fresh lemon or lime for flavor.

RULE NO. SIX:

Meals and snacks should not be stretched out. While you may occasionally linger over a relaxing meal, you should not multi-task or work while you eat.

RULE NO. SEVEN:

Finish your last meal or snack two to three hours before you go to sleep. During those two to three hours, do not eat or drink anything except black coffee, tea, herbal tea, water, or mineral water. You may add a squeeze of fresh lemon or lime for flavor.[1]

---

[1] If your prescription medications are to be taken at bedtime or taken with food or if you need to eat before bed to stabilize your blood sugar, you must follow your medical advice. It always takes precedence over plan rules.

PROPORTIONS

~   There is no portion control on the TQI diet and you should not count calories. You instead satisfy your body's appetite. You are not supposed to be hungry nor are you to eat more than you want. Your meals and snacks should be substantial enough to satisfy your appetite. When your are hungry, a snack may be as large as a dinner. When you are not hungry, a meal or snack may be as small as a single grape, a slice of apple, or a bite of a banana.

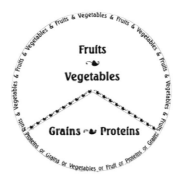

~   Lunch, dinner, and your two snacks must be proportional: At a minimum, two-thirds of every lunch, dinner, or snack must consist of fruits and/or vegetables. Protein and grain combined may not make up more than one-third of these meals.

~   Lunch, dinner, and your two snacks may consist entirely of vegetables and/or fruits.

~   You do not have to eat any protein at lunch, dinner, or your two snacks. However, you must have some form of protein for breakfast.

~   Grains are optional; you do not have to eat any grains at any meal or snack.

~   You must eat protein at breakfast, and breakfast should consist of one-third to one-half protein, and one-half to two-thirds vegetables or fruits. Do not eat grains for breakfast.

~   Potatoes and organic sprouted corn tortillas count as grains and may not be eaten for breakfast.

FOODS WE MAY EAT

- **Any vegetables**—fresh, frozen, or canned—as long as without added chemicals, additives or sweeteners.

- **Any fruits**—fresh, frozen, or canned—as long as without added chemicals, additives or sweeteners.

- **Any 100% whole grains** that are **not** relatives of wheat.

- **Any dried legumes,** dried beans, split peas, or lentils as well as products made from dried legumes. Any soybeans or soy products must be organic.

- **Any nuts, any seeds,** nut butter, or seed butter that is non-hydrogenated, and without added sugar or chemicals but no peanuts or peanut butter.

- **Any seafoods on the approved list.** (See p. 31.)

- **Any animal products on the approved list.** (See p. 31.)

- **Any cold pressed, non-deodorized oils** with the exception of corn, peanut, canola, cottonseed, and non-organic soybean oil.

- **Coconut milk** may be used to add flavor but is not to be drunk.

- **Unsweetened chocolate,** cocoa powder, cocoa nibs,[2] or whole cocoa beans.

- **Chicken, vegetable, or mushroom broth** if without added sugar.

- **Any herbs or spices,** except stevia or herb blends that have added sugar or chemicals.

- **Condiments made with approved foods,** such as salsas, mayonnaise, or mustard, made without added sugars.

- **Wheat-free organic soy or tamari sauce.**

- **Any vinegar** that does not contain coloring or sweeteners. Balsamic vinegars may be made from grape must.

---

[2] Make sure the cocoa beans or nibs are not coated in sweetened chocolate.

Foods that may be eaten freely on the elimination phase

Fruits

Apples	Apricots	Bananas	Blackberries
Blueberries	Cantaloupe	Clementines	Cranberries
Figs	Grapefruit	Grapes	Kiwi
Lemons	Limes	Mangoes	Melons
Oranges	Papayas	Peaches	Pears
Persimmons	Pineapple	Pomegranates	Plums

Vegetables

Artichokes	Arugula	Asparagus	Beans (green)
Bell peppers	Bok choy*	Broccoli*	Brussels sprouts*
Cabbage*	Cactus pads	Cauliflower*	Celery
Celery root	Chili peppers	Cucumber	Daikon*
Edamame	Eggplant	Endive	Escarole
Fennel	Garlic	Greens (any)	Jicama
Kohlrabi*	Leeks	Lettuce (any)	Mushrooms
Okra	Olives	Onions	Radicchio
Radishes*	Seaweed	Snow peas	Sprouts (not wheat)
Summer squash	Sweet corn	Tomatoes	Watercress*

Dried vegetables or mushrooms may be used in cooking.

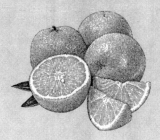

High-glycemic vegetables: Eat as desired but always with other foods.

Beets	Burdock	Carrots	Parsnips
Peas	Pumpkins	Rutabagas*	Sweet potatoes
Turnips*	Winter squash	Yams	

* Vegetables marked with a star (*) are cruciferous

FOODS THAT MAY BE EATEN FREELY ON THE ELIMINATION PHASE

Oils

Almond	Avocado	Coconut butter	Coconut milk
Coconut oil	Flaxseed	Grape seed	Macadamia nut
Olive, extra virgin	Palm fruit	Safflower	Sesame
Soybean, organic	Sunflower	Walnut	

Oils may not be solvent-extracted or hydrogenated. Safflower and sunflower oil are high in omega-6 fats and should be used sparingly. Olive oil must be the dominant oil in the diet.

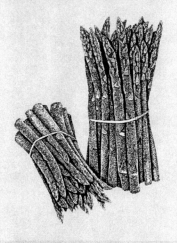

Other

Agar agar	Arrowroot	Chicken broth[1]	Chocolate[1]
Chutney[1]	Cocoa nibs[1]	Cocoa powder[1]	Coffee
Gomasio	Guar gum	Horseradish	Kelp powder
Kudzu	Pepper	Pomegranate concentrate/molasses	
Salsa[1]	Salt	Soy sauce, wheat-free	Spices, except stevia

Make sure items marked with a [1] are unsweetened.

FOODS ALWAYS EATEN PROPORTIONATELY
(Always with twice as many vegetables and/or fruits.)

Whole Grains

Amaranth	Black rice	Brown rice	Buckwheat (kasha)
Millet	Potatoes	Quinoa flakes	Quinoa flour
Red rice	Teff	Wild rice	

Any products (e.g., crackers) made from approved grains.

Legumes (protein)

Adzuki beans	Black beans	Chickpeas/Garbanzo beans	
Kidney beans	Lentils/Dahl	Navy beans	Pinto beans
Quinoa (whole, not flakes)	Soy milk[1]	Soy yoghurt[1]	Soy beans
Tempeh	Tofu	White beans	

Nuts and Seeds[2] (protein)

Almonds	Brazil nuts	Cashews	Chia seeds
Coconut, dried[1]	Filberts/Hazelnuts	Flaxseeds	Hemp seeds
Macadamia nuts	Pecans	Pine nuts	Pistachios
Pumpkin seeds	Sesame seeds	Soynuts, organic	Sunflower seeds
Walnuts			

Animal Products[3] (protein)

Anchovies	Arctic char	Chicken, skinless	Clams**
Cornish hens	Eggs	Halibut (Pacific)	Herring (Alaskan)
Lamb, grass-fed	Mackerel (Atlantic)	Mahi Mahi	Mussels**
Oysters**	Pollock (walleye)	Sablefish	Salmon (Alaskan)
Sardines	Shrimp (northern or pink)	Sole (rock)	Squid

Turkey, skinless

[1] These items must be unsweetened.
[2] Nuts and seeds may be raw, toasted, roasted, or salted as long as they are not processed in prohibited fats and do not contain added sugar or chemicals.
[3] Seafood must be wild unless marked with the symbols ** and *only* animal products included on the list are alllowed during the Elimination Phase.

FOODS NOT EATEN DURING THE ELIMINATION PHASE

Animal Products

Any seafood not listed on p. 31		Bacon	Beef
Bison/Buffalo	Butter	Buttermilk	Cheese
Chicken, cooked with skin on	Cottage cheese	Crab	Cream, sweet or sour
Cream cheese	Farmed fish	Farmed shrimp	Ghee
Half & Half	Ham	Lobster	Milk
Pork	Prawns	Processed meats	Sausage
Turkey, cooked with skin on	Tuna	Venison	Yoghurt

Dried Corn

Corn chips	Corn meal	Corn tortillas	Grits
Hominy	Polenta	Popcorn	Semolina

Any foods containing dried corn or dried corn products.

Sweeteners

Agave nectar	Anything with added sugar	Artificial sweeteners	Corn sweeteners
Corn syrup	Dried fruit	Evaporated cane juice	Fructose
Glycerin	High-fructose corn syrup	Honey	Jams, Jellies
Maltodextrin	Maple syrup	Molasses	Rice syrup
Sorbitol	Stevia	Succanat	Sugar, any type
Sugar alcohols	Syrup-packed fruit	Xylitol	

FOODS NOT EATEN DURING THE ELIMINATION PHASE

Wheat and Wheat Relatives

Barley	Beer	Bulgar	Couscous
Durum	Kamut	Malt, any type	Oats
Oat bran	Oat milk	Rye	Seitan
Spelt	Sprouted wheat	Triticale	Wheat
Wheat berries	Wheat bran	Wheat flour	Wheat germ
Wheat gluten	Wheat germ oil	Wheat starch	

Peanuts

Peanuts	Peanut butter

Oils

Canola oil	Corn oil	Cottonseed oil	Deodorized oils
Hydrogenated oils	Interesterified oils	Peanut oil	Solvent-extracted oils

Chemicals, Any

Additives	Artificial colors	Artificial fats	Artificial sweeteners
Flavorings, flavors	Modified starch	MSG	Preservatives

Other

Dried fruit	Fruit juice	Potato starch	Refined flour
Rice flour	Smoothies		

List of Natural Sweeteners

Agave nectar, barbados sugar, barley malt, beet sugar, blackstrap molasses, brown sugar, buttered syrup, cane crystals, cane juice crystals, cane sugar, caramel, carob syrup, castor sugar, confectioners' sugar, corn syrup, corn syrup solids, crystalline fructose, date sugar, demerara sugar, dextrin, dextran, dextrose, diastatic malt, diatase, D-mannose, evaporated cane juice, ethyl maltol, florida crystals, Free Flowing, fructose, fruit juice, fruit juice concentrate, galactose, glucose, glucose solids, glycerol, golden sugar, golden syrup, granulated sugar, grape sugar, grape juice concentrate, honey, icing sugar, invert sugar, lactose, malt syrup, maltose, maple syrup, molasses, muscovado sugar, organic raw sugar, panocha, powdered sugar, raw sugar, refiner's syrup, rice syrup, sorghum syrup, sucrose, sugar, syrup, table sugar, treacle, turbinado sugar, white sugar, yellow sugar.

List of Artificial Sweeteners

Acesulfame potassium, alitame, aspartame, aspartame-acesulfame salt, corn sweetener, cyclamate, equal, dextrin, dextran, dextrose, ethyl maltol, high-fructose corn syrup (HFCS, possibly corn sugar), isomalt, lactitol, maltitol, maltodextrin, mannitol, neohesperidine dihydrochalcone, neotame, nutrasweet, saccharin, sorbitol, splenda, sucralose, sugar twin, sunette, sweet one, sweet 'n low, sweet 'n safe, thaumatin, sylitol, E420, E421, E422, E950, E951, E952, E953, E954, E955, E956, E957, E959, E962, E965, E966, E967, E968.

List of Wheat and Wheat Relatives

There are many types of "true" wheat. Anything that bears the Latin name *Triticum* is a type of wheat: Bearded spring wheat (*Triticum aestivum*), beardless winter wheat (*Triticum hybernum*), rivet wheat (*Triticum turgidum*), einkorn wheat (*Triticum monococcum*), spelt (*Triticum spelta*), durum wheat (*Triticum durum*), farro or emmer wheat (*Triticum dicoccon*), and kamut (*Triticum turanicum*).

Other forms of wheat and wheat relatives to avoid include: Rye (*Secale cereale*), barley (*Hordeum vulgare*), bulgur, couscous, cracked wheat, cream of wheat, dextrose (may be derived from wheat), durum semolina, farina, most malts, oat bran, oat milk, oats (*Avena sativum*) in any form, sprouted wheat, wheat berries, wheat bran, wheat flour, wheat flour, wheat germ, wheat germ oil, wheat gluten (seitan), wheat pasta, wheat starch, and triticale.

List of Dairy Food

Bovine albumin, butter, butter fat, buttermilk, calcium caseinate, casein, cheese, condensed milk, cottage cheese, cream, curds, dairy, delactosed milk, evaporated milk, ghee, half & half, hydrolyzed casein, hydrolyzed milk protein, ice cream, ice milk, kefir, Kosher symbol "D," lactaid milk, lactalbumin, lacteeze milk, lactoglobulin, lactose free milk, milk, milk fat, milk formula, milk solid, pasteurized milk, raw milk, recaldent (milk casein derivative used in some gums), rennet casein, skim milk, sodium caseinate, sour cream, sour milk, whey, whey protein, whipping cream, yoghurt.

PRINCIPLES TO EAT BY

- ❧ Eat lots of berries—the wilder the berry, the better.

- ❧ Eat as many and as many different types of vegetables as possible.

- ❧ Eat more cruciferous vegetables[3] (marked with a * in the table of vegetables.)

- ❧ Enjoy high-glycemic vegetables (see p. 29) but do not eat them alone; always combine them with other foods.

- ❧ Eat garlic and onions often.

- ❧ Season your food with herbs and spices.

- ❧ Olive oil should be your main cooking oil. For occasional high-temperature cooking, use coconut or non–solvent extracted grape seed or avocado oil.

- ❧ Eat a variety of nuts and/or seeds.

- ❧ Do not drink your food. Avoid juices or smoothies. Use nut, soy, rice, or other "milks" to add flavor but not as stand-alone drinks. Count these "milks," either as protein (nut or soy) or grain (rice). Make sure they do not contain added sugar or canola oil. Do not use "grain milks" at breakfast.

- ❧ Eat good fats and make sure olive oil is the primary fat in your diet. Limit your saturated animal fats and fats high in omega-6 fats, such as safflower and sunflower oil.

- ❧ Read labels carefully. Processed, packaged, and prepared foods often contain chemicals, added sugars, wheat, corn, corn derivatives, and canola oil.

- ❧ Proteins and grains must always be eaten with fruits or vegetables; they are never eaten by themselves.

---

[3] Those with intestinal issues may find these vegetables difficult to digest. If something does not agree with you, do not eat it. But try them again at some point later on as you may find they eventually agree with you.

REMINDER
FOODS TO AVOID DURING THE ELIMINATION PHASE:

❀   Sweeteners including added sweeteners and artificial sweeteners.

❀   Wheat in any form, including sprouted wheat, all wheat relatives, and all wheat derivatives.

❀   Dairy, including goat cheese, ghee, and butter.

❀   Dried corn in any form.

❀   Peanuts in any form including peanut butter, peanut oil, and any food containing peanuts.

❀   Corn, peanut, cottonseed, canola, hydrogenated, trans-fat, solvent extracted, and non-organic soybean oils.

❀   Any animal product not on the approved list. (See p. 31.)

❀   Chemicals and heavily processed foods.

❀   Non-organic soy and soy products.

❀   Refined grains, including rice flour and potato starch.

❀   Alcoholic beverages.

❀   Juices, smoothies, and other "food beverages."

❀   Dried fruit, including dates.

❀   Avoid foods you have been told you may be sensitive to.

CHAPTER FOUR

Overview of Plan Principles

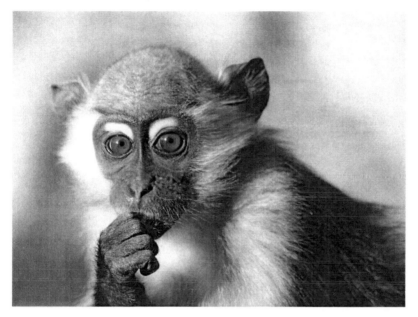

Reflecting on the reasons for the rules.

The approved foods and the principles that govern how we eat on the TQI diet are explained in detail in the chapters that follow. These foods are rich in vitamins and antioxidants, good plant fats, high-quality protein, and other nutrients we need to quiet inflammation and be healthy. The foods that are emphasized are especially rich in anti-inflammatory and liver-protective compounds.

MEALS AND SNACKS

1. THERE IS NO PORTION CONTROL

On the TQI diet, there is no limit on the amount of food we may eat nor is there a minimum amount we must eat. We do not count calories and we do not monitor portion sizes. Instead, we focus entirely on eating the right foods in the right proportions at the right times. This is what quiets inflammation and, as we get healthier, our body moves toward a healthy weight without us having to fret over calories. Often, as we provide consistent nutrients to our body, our appetite naturally decreases. It may be that we are drawn to overeat bad foods (e.g., pizzas, fast food burgers, ice cream, etc.) in a near-futile attempt to get all of the nutrients we need from those nutrient-deficient foods.

2. PROPORTIONATE MEALS

The proportionate meal is a key feature of the TQI diet. Instead of counting calories or measuring portions, we make sure that we eat proportionately. The importance of proportions will be explained in many different ways in coming chapters and will not be explained at this point. Here we will simply cover how to apply the rule: Lunch, dinner, and both snacks must be proportionate.[1] Proportionate means that at least two-thirds of lunch, dinner, and

---

[1] Different rules apply to breakfast, see p. 45.

the two snacks must consist of fruits or vegetables. The other one-third may consist of any mixture of grains, proteins, fruits, and/or vegetables that suit you in the moment.

In other words, you might choose to have a meal consisting of:

One-third fish (counts as protein) and two-thirds vegetables.

You might have a meal of one-third brown rice (counts as grain) with one-third vegetables and one-third fruit.

Another meal might consist of one-sixth baked tofu (protein) with one-sixth brown rice pasta (grain) and two-thirds vegetables.

Another night, you might choose to have soup and salad with some fruit. (All fruit and vegetable).

A snack might consist of an apple (all fruit) or an avocado with salsa (all vegetable) or a handful of nuts (one-third protein) with two handfuls of grapes (two-thirds fruit).

For the most part, we gauge proportions visually, by looking at our plate. On other occasions, if more practical, we measure by volume: If we grab a handful of nuts (protein) or crackers (grain), we simply grab two handfuls of fruit or vegetables to balance them. If we have a cup of quinoa (protein), we balance it with two cups of green salad (vegetable).

We measure the food in the form that we eat it: If we are eating uncooked chard—or less likely—raw rice or unpopped popcorn, we measure the food that way. On the other hand, if we have cooked the rice and chard, and popped the popcorn, we measure it that way. There is no need to weigh or actually measure the components on our plate. Over the long run the proportions will be accurate even if slightly off in the moment. But, be aware that we often play games with ourselves. The goal is to increase our intake of fruits and vegetables, not to push the limits and find ways to eat more protein and grain. When in doubt err on the side of eating more fruits and vegetables.[2]

---

[2] Interestingly, people tend to want to measure their chard and popcorn raw even though they are eating them cooked/popped. This allows them to eat more protein with their chard and less fruit with their popcorn. Our goal is to overcome our almost universal tendency to avoid eating much in the way of vegetables.

Eating proportionate meals allows you to continue making many of your favorite dishes even if they are not proportionate in and of themselves. Simply add sides of vegetables to make the overall meal proportionate. For instance, if a chicken curry you love is heavy on protein and light on vegetables, all you need do is to make sure that your vegetable side dish(es) bring your meal back into balance.

The proportionate meal is dramatically different from the way most of us have been eating. The Western diet tends to make concentrated forms of protein the centerpiece of the meals and uses vegetables more as condiments or sides. As you begin to eat proportionate meals, it may be easier to first plate your vegetables and then figure out how much protein or grain to add to balance your meal. If you plate the protein first, you may end up with a bigger meal than you wish to eat. Or, more common, you will eat all the protein but not finish the vegetables and end up not eating proportionately. This will cease being an issue as you become more accustomed to eating vegetables and learn how to prepare them in more exciting ways: Eventually vegetables will become the centerpiece of your plate and your protein and grain become the accents and condiments.

3. EAT THREE MEALS AND TWO SNACKS DAILY

It is important to get all of the nutrients we need on a regular and consistent basis. Eating healthy meals and snacks regularly ensures this happens. If we are to reduce food cravings it is also important to make sure that we are not hungry.

Although many people have trouble eating three meals a day, let alone adding two snacks, it is important to work all of these meals and snacks in over the day. Many of us are "mind driven," we often focus on our tasks at hand without taking the time to eat. Perhaps we are not hungry but it is equally likely that we simply are too busy. During the Elimination Phase, we are going to regularly check in with our body to see if it needs nutrients, even if we are not interested in taking the time to eat. It is entirely possible that some extra antioxidants might help counter the toxic chemicals and oxidative stress that may be part of our day.

Snacks are also important because our livers may not maintain our blood sugar levels very well between meals. If we go too long without food, we experience blood sugar lows that can cause headaches, jitteriness, fatigue, or cravings for sugary food. Frequent and regular meals and snacks make it easier for the liver to maintain our blood sugar levels. This makes it easier for us to stay on the diet.

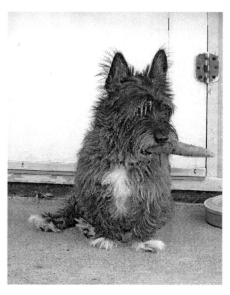

Snacks are mandatory.

Remember, if eating snacks is a struggle: Snacks (and meals) may be as small or large as you wish. A grape if you are not hungry, a dinner-sized serving if you are ravenous.

After you have eaten well for a number of months and have successfully quieted inflammation, you may choose to eliminate snacks if you find that you are not hungry; but initially it is important to eat all meals and snacks.

4. Eat a healthy breakfast soon after rising

It is crucial to begin the day with a good breakfast. Each night as we sleep, the body repairs itself. This repair process uses up the body's store of amino acids, antioxidants, vitamins, and other nutrients. We wake up depleted and, unless we replenish lost nutrients, we are not able to carry ourselves through the day in a healthy fashion. Lacking necessary building blocks, we either "borrow" needed nutrients from "less important" parts of the body (such as our muscles) or we forego needed repairs until we eventually eat. Over the long term, this is hard on and damaging to the body.

We should wake up with an appetite and our first meal should rebuild our stores of the depleted compounds. That is why we eat something almost immediately after getting up. It is why our breakfast consists of foods with concentrated amounts of protein combined with fruits and vegetables with a target ratio of one-third to one-half protein, with the remainder consisting of fruits and vegetables. The proteins replenish our stores of free amino acids (see chapter 16). The fruits and vegetables provide needed antioxidants, vitamins, and other phytonutrients.

Grains do not contain any nutrients missing from our fruits and vegetables; they do, however, provide some sugars and fats that we do not need. We all have an over-abundance of omega-6 fats, and should not start our day with the omega-6 fats found in grains (see chapter 6). Furthermore, studies show that people who begin their day with grains tend to experience more cravings for sugars and other "inappropriate" foods later in the day. These cravings make it harder to stay on a healthy diet. In contrast, most people report that adding protein and good fats at breakfast gives them a more even and sustained energy level throughout the day.

If you usually start your day by engaging in relatively strenuous athletic activity, your breakfast may be small: Some nuts and a little fresh fruit, or sliced apple with nut butter before you work out. This will not hamper your activity but instead will support your ability to exercise. Back from your exercise, immediately have a snack that looks more like a substantial breakfast.[3] This snack

---

[3]   After exercise, the body is primed to replace glycogen stores in the muscles. It is important to eat within a half hour of demanding exercise and to eat foods that provide glucose. A post-workout meal should consist of high-glycemic vegetables and high-carbohydrate foods (e.g., baked garnet yams and brown rice cakes) with some protein to help replenish glycogen. If you do not do this, you may find your endurance dropping.

may be large but should follow the Rule of Proportions. The same holds true for those who cannot stomach the thought of breakfast, especially a breakfast that includes protein. Start off with a small meal of nuts and fruit eaten soon after rising. Then in late morning have a larger snack that is more of a complete breakfast, still focusing on protein, fruits, and vegetables rather than grains.

Most of us are used to a very different breakfast consisting primarily of grains. We either have toast and coffee or a more substantial breakfast of granola or oatmeal. Abandoning our familiar grains can seem overwhelming at first. The change seems even more difficult because we may be leaving our cozy bed to head off to stress-filled jobs and activities. Often, we eat breakfast foods that trigger an adrenalin release, to "jump-start" the day. Sugars, refined carbohydrates, caffeine, and foods we are sensitive to cause a flow of adrenalin that momentarily boosts our energy. Unfortunately, the energy gain is short-lived and the subsequent drop in energy makes us want more of those same foods. As you embark on this eating plan, you may miss your morning adrenalin boost,[4] but you will soon experience the sustainable energy a good breakfast provides. There are many simple and satisfying breakfasts available and we rapidly become very fond of a supportive morning meal. Hang in there!

5. Breakfast proportions

The breakfast proportions differ slightly from those of other meals. Our breakfast consists of one-third to one-half protein with the remainder a mixture of fruits and/or vegetables. We eat no grains for breakfast. We use breakfast to replenish stores of nutrients depleted over night. Some concentrated type of protein is required at breakfast in order to restore our pool of amino acids. To accomplish this goal, we may eat slightly more protein than at other meals. We also eat fruits and vegetables to help us metabolize

---

[4] The main reason people find the change in breakfast challenging is because the new breakfast choices are not inflammatory to the body and they do not cause a release of adrenalin the way wheat, sugar, and dairy do. Many initially miss the "zip" their old breakfast provided. However, their bodies do not and instead soon thrive on the change.

that protein properly. We do not eat grains. At other meals and snacks, concentrated protein is optional and grain is allowed.

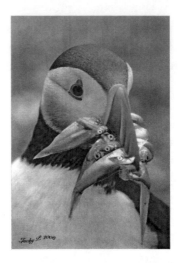

Protein is an important part of breakfast.

6. WE DO NOT GRAZE

We eat regularly (breakfast, lunch, dinner, and two snacks). In between meals and snacks we do not eat anything because food, including no-calorie artificial sweeteners, may trigger the release of insulin. To avoid this potential release, we do not put "whiteners" in our beverages, we do not chew gum or suck on breath mints; we do not eat at all except at meals and snack times.

In our culture, we often graze. We drink coffee with milk and sugar throughout the morning, we have a few grapes here and there, and we sample foods while shopping. Every time we eat, we secrete some insulin; if we eat constantly, we are constantly in an "insulin state." This is detrimental because we have other metabolic hormones that do not get an opportunity to come into play if too much insulin is present. Not grazing (having periods when we do not eat) helps break the insulin dominance in our body and allows these other hormones to work. This helps restore a hormonal rhythm that most of our bodies have lost (see chapter 9). Eating constantly also contributes to leptin resistance, a problem that tends to prevent the body from losing weight (see chapter 10).

On this plan, we may add soy or nut milk to our morning coffee but when we leave the breakfast table, we leave our whitened coffee on the table and we do not eat again until snack time. We may drink black coffee, unwhitened tea, herbal teas, mineral water, and water between meals and snacks. These beverages may be flavored with a squeeze of fresh lemon or lime, or some herbs but no other fruit or fruit flavors.

We also avoid stretching our meals out by working in between bites of food. If we do not limit the length of our meals, we end up grazing over the course of the day. This jeopardizes our ability to bring other hormones into play. For more information, see FAQ page 214.

7. WE DO NOT EAT BEFORE BED

We stop eating altogether two to three hours before going to sleep. There are two main reasons for this rule; they have to do with growth hormone and leptin cycles.

Growth hormone

Once we reach our adult height, we produce much less growth hormone. As adults, we have one predictable daily burst of growth hormone that occurs a few hours after we fall asleep. This growth hormone burst is important because it helps maintain our muscle mass as we age. However, we only release growth hormone on nights when we do not eat and secrete insulin in the hours immediately before sleep. If we eat a bedtime snack, the insulin released will shut down the important burst of growth hormone that night. Shutting down growth hormone on a regular basis makes it difficult to maintain muscle mass.[5]

Leptin cycles

The second reason for adults to give up bedtime snacks involves the hormone leptin. Our fat cells use leptin to communicate with the brain about our energy stores. When fat stores are high, fat cells secrete more leptin. In response, the brain turns down

---

[5] Growing children produce growth hormone throughout the day and night. They may eat more than two snacks, including a bedtime snack if they are hungry—and the snack is healthy (see p. 204).

appetite and turns up our metabolism because we can "afford" to burn fat. When fat stores are low, less leptin is produced, and the brain turns up appetite and turns down metabolism so our energy stores will last longer.

Leptin has a daily cycle of waxing and waning in addition to bursts in response to periodic changes in the body's fat stores. In a healthy person, leptin levels begin to rise in the evening and, as levels rise, appetite decreases. Leptin reaches a peak at about bedtime (as long as we are not on a starvation diet) when appetite should be nonexistent. This natural waning of appetite happens because we are not nocturnal creatures and should not have food cravings right before going to sleep.

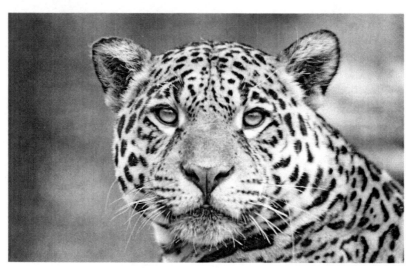

Nocturnal animals hunt and eat at night.

Picture one of our hunter/gatherer ancestors living in a jungle: Panthers, jaguars, and other carnivores see in the dark; humans do not. There are venomous snakes and spiders about that cannot be seen in the dark. The waters are filled with piranhas and caymans, and the logs across the waters are slippery and near impossible to traverse in the dark. Night is a dangerous time for humans; it is not the time to go looking for a bedtime snack. Our species' ability to survive was enhanced by not experiencing hunger at night; only nocturnal creatures should eat at night.

Then, as the night progresses, leptin levels begin to decline. As dawn approaches, the brain turns up the appetite and turns down metabolism in response to the drop in leptin levels. This triggers a desire to eat breakfast. The slowed metabolism conserves fat stores to ensure the hunter/gatherer does not run out of steam before finding a suitable breakfast. In summary, humans should not be hungry at night and should be quite hungry in the morning.

Yet many of us have exactly the opposite hunger pattern. No matter how large our dinner, no matter how much extra fat we have stored on our body, we crave something to eat before bed. Then, overnight we deplete the nutrients in our body but nonetheless wake without an appetite for breakfast. At most we want a jolt of caffeine and maybe some bread but we are not interested in foods that supply needed nutrients. Our leptin clocks are out of order.

When we eat before bed, we secrete insulin. Insulin shuts down growth hormone. However, it cannot shut off leptin's daily rhythm. Instead, it shifts leptin's "clock" and we begin to experience hunger and satiety at the "wrong" times of the day. As we give up our bedtime snacks, we begin to reset our leptin clock back to where it was intended to be.

There is an additional side benefit to resetting the leptin clock. Leptin's daily rhythm is tied to another hormone, melatonin. Melatonin controls how well we sleep and in some respects how "awake" we feel during the day. As our leptin clock shifts, melatonin's does as well. If our melatonin clock is "off," we have less melatonin during the night when we should be sleeping and more during the day when we should be wide awake. As we give up bedtime snacks, people typically quickly report that they are sleeping better and feel more clearheaded during the day.

8. Why potatoes and sprouted corn tortillas count as grain

Potatoes are vegetables that contain some valuable nutrients. However, they are a high-glycemic vegetable and a vegetable we tend to overeat to the exclusion of more nutritious vegetables. They are counted as grain to prevent us from overeating them. Sprouted corn tortillas are made from dried corn, a grain, and are counted as such. The reason why that form of dried corn is allowed during the Elimination Phase is explained on page 223.

RESTRICT CERTAIN FOODS DURING THE ELIMINATION PHASE

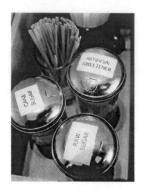 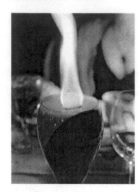

Sugars are inflammatory.

1. AVOID ALL NATURAL, ADDED, AND ARTIFICIAL SWEETENERS

Natural sweeteners

There are many plant-derived sweeteners ranging from white, brown, and powdered sugar to honey, maple syrup, and molasses. While there are differences among them, at their core they are all the same—a mixture of fructose and glucose. We need to limit them because all sugars are inherently inflammatory.

The glucose in these natural sweeteners raises our blood sugar levels quickly and causes our insulin levels to rise quickly. This creates many problems for the body and is reason enough to avoid sugars (see chapter 9). Sweeteners deplete our stores of magnesium in the liver. Most of us need more, not less, magnesium if we are to quiet inflammation (see chapter 12). Additionally, sweeteners cause oxidative stress which damages the body (see chapter 7).

None of the sweeteners provide any significant amount of nutrients.[6] However, because their taste pleases us, sugars play a prominent role in the Western diet. If we are to willingly limit their presence, we must acknowledge the many negative effects of sweeteners and become disciplined about avoiding sweetened foods. A list of various sugars is provided on page 34.

---

[6] While less-processed sweeteners (such as organic raw sugar, honey, or maple syrup) have a few more beneficial components than refined sugar, from the body's perspective, they are *all* ultimately an inflammatory mixture of glucose and fructose.

Added, or the often overlooked, sweeteners

In order to quiet inflammation, it is critical to avoid all sweeteners during the Elimination Phase. Many people think they have eliminated sugar by avoiding obvious sweets but fail to realize how many other foods in their diet contain added sugar. Much of our sugar intake comes from eating prepared foods with added sugar. In fact, the average American eats 20 teaspoons of added sugar a day.

We need to read the entire ingredient label on the foods we buy if we want to avoid added sweeteners. And we need to stop excusing ourselves when we eat foods with "hidden" (or added) sugar—"it is just a teaspoon in my coffee," "sugar is the last ingredient in the catsup," "I just put a dab of jam in the salad dressing," "I'm sure they did not put too much sugar on the sweet potato fries," etc. If we avoid added sugars, so overly abundant in our foods, we will be able to choose occasionally to have fabulous desserts after finishing the Elimination and Testing Phases (see chapter 22).

To effectively eliminate added sugar from our diet, we must distinguish between a food label's *ingredient* list and its *nutrition* facts. The ingredient list tells us what ingredients the manufacturer put in the product; the nutrition facts reveal the calories and nutritional content of one serving of those ingredients. Make a habit of carefully reading the ingredient list of any foods you are thinking of buying. Make sure no prohibited sweeteners (natural or artificial) are on this list. (See p. 34.)

Even though sugar should not be on the ingredient list, it may, however, be listed on the nutrition label. Why? Because many foods are naturally sweet and contain some form of natural (not added) sugar. Fruits contain sugar in the form of fructose, as do some sweet vegetables. Thus, the nutrition label for these foods will list an amount of sugar contained in a serving of that food. The fructose, however, is naturally occurring and is not added by the manufacturer, so no sugar is listed on the ingredient list.

For example, the ingredient list for canned corn should only contain corn, water, and perhaps some salt. There should be no mention of sucrose, fructose, splenda, or maltodextrin. In contrast, the canned corn's nutrition label will list a certain amount of sugar—those are the natural sugars present in the corn kernels that make them taste pleasantly sweet.

In summary: Natural sugars found in whole foods are fine but added sugar in any form is eliminated.

Artificial sweeteners

There are many artificial (or man-made) sweeteners present in our diet. We favor artificial sweeteners because they taste sweet but they do not contain calories nor do they raise blood sugar levels. Because they are calorie free, we see artificial sweeteners as "diet" or "weight-loss" aids. Ironically, artificial sweeteners make fattening foods sound less fattening, because they are "sugar free." The wide acceptance of these compounds as "weight-loss" helpers depends on the misperception that sugar is the sole, or the main, cause of obesity and health problems. Sugar does play a big role in obesity, but the artificial sweetener manufacturers vastly overplay its role.

When we use artificial sweeteners, we are trying to trick our bodies. We hope to be able to eat sweet-tasting foods without paying a price for them. However, life does not work that way—or at least our bodies do not work that way. When we taste something sweet, we immediately send a signal to the brain that we are eating something sweet. The brain anticipates, quite reasonably, that our blood sugar will soon rise so it tells the pancreas to begin secreting insulin. Our insulin levels rise, but our blood sugar does not. The insulin causes our blood sugar levels to drop somewhat, which in turn triggers cravings for foods to get our blood sugar back up where it belongs. Animals fed artificial sweeteners gain weight because the sweeteners induce them to eat more. On this plan, we avoid artificial sweeteners because they trigger cravings for inflammatory foods and cause weight gain.

Another reason to avoid artificial sweeteners is that they taste intensely sweet, far sweeter than anything natural. They make our fruits and vegetables taste bland in comparison. Without these sweeteners in our diets, real food tastes sweeter and far more enjoyable.

Finally, we avoid all artificial sweeteners because they are either man-made chemicals or are heavily processed. They have a variety of effects in our bodies. Experts disagree about whether these sweeteners are harmful. Many scientists and nutritionists claim that they have substantial negative side effects. No one claims that they are good for us. Given their lack of benefit and potential detriment, we eliminate them.

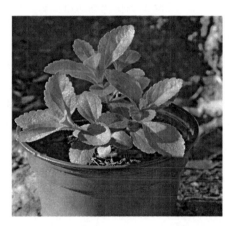

Stevia, an herbal sweetener.

Stevia is an herb, a natural product, that is gaining in popularity as a substitute for artificial sweeteners. It has a similar effect in our body: It tastes very sweet but does not affect our blood sugar levels. It does not provide calories. It generates the same reaction in the body: A release of insulin that lowers blood sugar levels that in turn often triggers food cravings. The only difference is that stevia does not appear to directly harm the body the way chemicals may. But for this latter fact, stevia poses all the same problems as artificial sweeteners, so we eliminate stevia as well. Occasionally, high-fructose corn syrup, the corn-derived sweetener maltodextrin, and most sugar alcohols (such as xylitol) are classified as "natural." Because they are heavily processed and manipulated compounds, we treat them as artificial sweeteners.

2. ELIMINATE ALL FORMS OF WHEAT

Gluten is a group of wheat proteins that is present in all members of the wheat family. It triggers a severe inflammatory reaction in people with celiac disease. It also causes a milder inflammatory reaction in many others who do not have celiac disease. In addition, people without any known sensitivities to wheat may produce inflammatory cytokines after eating wheat. Adverse reactions to wheat are very common, and much more frequent than for any other grain. It is such a common problem food that the government requires labels to specifically state if there are even traces of wheat present in a food. Gluten-like proteins found in rye and barley (close relatives of wheat) also may trigger inflammatory responses. Oats, even though a more distant relative of wheat than rye or barley, can also trigger inflammatory reactions, either because the oat crop is contaminated with wheat (a fairly common event) or because the oat protein avenin is perceived by the immune system as substantially similar to one of the gluten proteins.

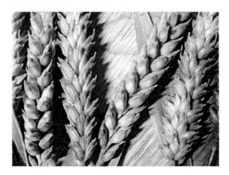
Wheat spikes.

During the Elimination Phase, all members of the wheat family are off-limits. Sprouted wheat products are also eliminated. Sprouting the wheat seeds transforms some, but not all, of the gluten. Because some gluten is present, sprouted grains may trigger mild inflammation. Sometimes claims are made that certain types of wheat do not cause the adverse reaction that "true" wheat does. Unfortunately, there is little substance to these claims. For instance, kamut is said to be an ancient Egyptian strain of wheat unlikely to cause a "wheat reaction." In fact, it is a fairly recent hybrid of wheat and contains gluten. Both spelt and farro are often marketed as well tolerated by people with a wheat sensitivity. As a rule, they do contain less gluten than other wheat varieties, but both still have enough gluten to cause reactions. Buckwheat (*Fagopyrum esculantum*), however, is not a wheat relative and may be eaten despite the fact that its common name makes it sound as if it is related to wheat.

We will test our individual reactions to wheat in the Testing Phase. If you do not react adversely to wheat, it will be added back to your regular diet. However, in order to do this testing, we must first eliminate all wheat for at least three weeks while eating a diet that quiets inflammation.

3. Eliminate dairy

Dairy is a problem food for many people for two main reasons: Some individuals lack an enzyme needed to digest milk while others experience an inflammatory response to milk proteins.[7] Occasionally, individuals react only to cow's milk products and not other dairy (such as goat or sheep) but, more often, if there is a sensitivity, it extends to all milk products, whether cow, goat, or sheep.

First, some individuals do not make the enzyme, lactase, that breaks down milk sugar (lactose). This condition is known as lactose intolerance. Individuals who are lactose intolerant experience diarrhea and digestive upset whenever they eat dairy. This problem can be avoided by taking a lactase enzyme supplement or by only eating specially prepared lactose-free dairy. The fact that someone cannot digest dairy without help suggests that it is not a food they are designed to eat. However, lactose intolerance is not a food sensitivity.

Second, many people experience an inflammatory reaction to one or more milk proteins. Sensitivity to the proteins lactalbumin and casein are the most common. Those who are sensitive to casein tend to react to all types of dairy. Those who are sensitive to lactalbumin sometimes can tolerate goat or sheep dairy, but not cow dairy products (or the other way around). This is possible because the structure of lactalbumin varies from species to species, and some immune systems can distinguish between them.

---

[7] It is possible to be both lactose intolerant and sensitive to dairy proteins.

Often individuals happily report that they react to milk but do quite well with cheese or yoghurt. This is usually simply a case of an inflammatory response "flying under the radar." In fact, the yoghurt or cheese do ignite an inflammatory response in these cases as they too contain the troublesome milk proteins. In the case of yoghurt, the inflammatory response is subdued (but not eliminated) because the beneficial bacterial strains in the yoghurt somewhat calm the immune system. Reactions to cheese often go unnoticed in part because we tend to eat smaller amounts of cheese at any given time. Cheeses also contain a much higher percentage fat and thus contain proportionately less of the troublesome protein than milk does, but still have enough to excite the immune system. Additionally, many individuals are so fond of cheese that they simply ignore that cheese may cause any negative response in their body.

Other problems with dairy include that it may be produced using genetically modified bovine growth hormone and the cows may be fed genetically modified corn feed (see chapter 20). Many of the dairy products in the marketplace come from factory-farmed animals. This method of farming results in dairy products higher in omega-6 fats (see chapter 6). Also, because cows are high on the food chain, dairy products deliver persistent toxins, often estrogenic in nature (see chapter 8). Moreover, dairy contains no fiber and thus does not feed our beneficial intestinal flora (see chapter 5). Finally, dairy is an acidic food from the viewpoint of our kidneys, liver, and bones and is taxing to these systems (see chapter 16).

We will test our individual reactions to dairy in the Testing Phase. If you do not react adversely to dairy, it returns as a food choice. However, to be able to test, we must first eliminate all dairy for at least three weeks while eating foods that quiet inflammation.

4. ELIMINATE DRIED CORN

Corn generally comes as fresh or "sweet" corn and as dried corn. These are different varieties of corn and are used quite differently. Far more dried corn is grown: Of the eight billion bushels of corn grown each year, less than one percent is fresh corn.

Dried corn has a heavy presence in the Western diet because so many ingredients made from dried corn are used in processed and fast foods. This is a real problem for those with true corn allergies because it is extremely difficult to avoid corn while eating any processed food. For instance, about 15% of the dried corn crop is turned into things like alcohol, oil, starch, corn syrup, and dextrose. All of these may contain enough corn protein to cause allergic reactions in highly sensitive individuals. Corn oil is often used as a commercial frying oil, in salad dressings, and it is often an ingredient in margarine. Cornstarch is used to thicken and stabilize other ingredients, and shows up in baking powder, prepared mixes, candies, baking goods, and puddings. Corn syrup replaces sugar in bakery and dairy products, sweet beverages, candies, ketchup, pickles, and other condiments. High-fructose corn syrup (HFCS) and dextrose are found in candies, baked foods, table syrup, sweet beverages, ketchup, pickles, and other condiments. Corn grits are used to brew beers and ales, to make corn flakes, or are eaten as is. Corn meal, with its long shelf life, is used to make breads, snack foods (corn chips and tacos), ready-to-eat breakfast cereals, and polenta.

Dried corn is also found in unexpected places. Corn oil is found in some toothpastes, and some brands contain enough corn protein to trigger a reaction in extremely sensitive people. Corn syrup is used as a texturizer and carrying agent in cosmetics. Adhesives for envelopes, stamps, and stickers may contain corn starch. Medication can also be a source of hidden corn. People with corn allergies need to be leery of any food containing baking powder, caramel color, confectioners' sugar, dextrin, dextrose, fructose, hominy, invert sugar, invert syrup, lactic acid, maltodextrins, manitol, sorbitol, starch, vanilla extract, vegetable broth, and vegetable starch.

The prevalence of true corn allergies in our population is difficult to track down. Fortunately, corn sensitivities (which concern us) seem to be fairly uncommon. However, dried corn can nonetheless be inflammatory because it is a food higher in omega-6 fats, and because we consume, directly and indirectly, too much corn. Additionally, dried corn is quite susceptible to

Aspergillus flavus, a mold also often found on peanuts (see p. 246). Many of us are sensitive to molds and thus may react periodically when we eat dried corn.

During the Elimination Phase, we avoid all dried corn. This significantly reduces the amount of corn in our diet, even though we continue to eat fresh corn and sprouted corn tortillas. Then, in the Testing Phase, we measure our individual response to adding back dried corn to the diet. If this does not trigger an inflammatory reaction, we can eat all forms of whole corn (as opposed to corn-based chemicals) in moderation, if we remember that it is a grain, must be eaten in the right proportions, and not eaten at breakfast.

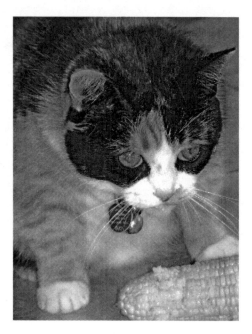

Sweet corn is a popular vegetable.

Of course, if you prove to be sensitive to corn, you need to quit eating all corn, including fresh and sprouted corn.

5. ELIMINATE PEANUTS

Although they are called nuts, peanuts belong to the pea family. Peanuts grow underground; nuts grow on trees. Because peanuts grow underground, they are very susceptible to a variety of molds. *Aspergillus flavus* is a mold that grows on peanuts. This mold thrives on foods dried and stored in humid climates, and peanuts are the crop most likely to be contaminated with it. (Dried corn is the second most likely.) *Aspergillus* is a particular problem because it makes a toxin, aflatoxin B, that is a strong liver carcinogen.

The aflatoxin content of our food is monitored by the government but is not possible to entirely avoid. Nonetheless, we should do what we can. Thus, peanuts and peanut butter once opened, should be refrigerated to limit the production of aflatoxin B. The potential presence of mold also creates a dilemma in terms of choosing between organic and conventional peanut products. The former are not treated with fungicides and may, theoretically, be more likely to host molds (although there is no evidence that this is the case). The alternative is to choose non-organic products that typically are treated with very toxic fungicides, posing other problems, especially for children.

Another problem with peanuts is simply that we tend to overeat them. True peanut allergies are very common today, and are on the rise in the U.S. They are much less common in other countries where people eat fewer peanuts, less peanut oil, and less peanut butter. Fortunately, peanut sensitivities are uncommon. We instead avoid peanuts during the Elimination Phase to reduce our exposure to molds as well as to motivate us to explore a greater variety of other nuts and seeds.[8] This reduces our tendency to favor peanuts a bit too much. We test our individual sensitivity to peanuts during the Testing Phase. Of course, if you are allergic to peanuts, you will not test them.

6. Oils to eliminate

Hydrogenated and deodorized vegetable oils

Many of the oils in our food have been deodorized (heated to high temperatures to improve shelf life) or manipulated in other ways. Those processes create chemical bonds—such as trans-

---

[8] For most, this is a beneficial change because nuts and seeds are rich in good fats and other nutritious compounds. However, sensitivities to tree nuts are also common and are therefore included in Plateau Testing (chapter 23).

fat bonds—that the body cannot properly digest. To protect our health, we avoid any oils that are refined, deodorized, and/or hydrogenated.

Corn and peanut oil

Oils from corn and peanuts are removed during the Elimination Phase as part of eliminating corn and peanuts. We especially benefit from removing corn oil, a cheap, often poorly made oil that tends to predominate in processed foods and adds significant amounts of omega-6 fats to our diet.

Cottonseed oil

Cotton is a plant used to make clothes. It is not a food. Cottonseed oil is not a good food either. It lowers sperm counts in male animals and may have negative reproductive effects in both men and women. It is used as a food oil mostly because it is inexpensive. In addition, cotton is a heavily sprayed crop, and will often carry greater amounts of pesticides into the oil.[9]

Canola oil

We are taught that canola oil is a very healthy oil, and canola has a strong lobby promoting its sales. It is a very common ingredient in our food. Aspects of canola, however, are troublesome.

The "rape plant" (*Brassica campestris*) produces canola oil. This plant's oil was historically used as a heating and lighting oil rather than as a food oil because rapeseed contained a high percentage of a toxic compound, erucic acid. Erucic acid can cause fatty degeneration of the heart and adrenals. In the early 1970s, the rape plant was hybridized to create a variety that produced much, much less erucic acid.[10] The oil's name was changed from rapeseed oil

---

[9] Cotton is cultivated on about 2.5 percent of the earth's surface. Around 16 percent of all insecticides are used on that cotton, including some of the most toxic types.

[10] Many pro-canola websites describe its hybridization as very natural. In fact, it was done using modern techniques which involve radiating the plant and then selecting seeds created by that mutagenic event—a far cry from "old" techniques. Moreover, hybrids have been created that are purposely low in omega-3 fats to prevent the oil from going rancid but significantly reducing its health benefits. http://www.canolacouncil.org/chapter2.aspx

to canola oil to make it easier to market.[11] Government agencies concluded that as long as the erucic acid content of the oil was below two to three percent, the oil was not unhealthy.

We eliminate canola oil because our goal is not simply to avoid things that are unhealthy. We need to go beyond that and place an emphasis on eating foods that are good for us. Compare olive and canola oil: Olive oil has been a food for millennia and virtually all studies show it provides significant health benefits. In contrast, canola oil has been a food for less than half a century and the government has concluded that it is not harmful to us. We are going to use the healthful olive oil rather than ingesting even small amounts of erucic acid.[12]

Non-organic soybean oil

Most conventionally grown soybeans are genetically modified (GM). In order to avoid GM foods, we avoid non-organic soybean oil. In addition, any organic soybean oil used should be unrefined.

7. Eliminate some animal products

We narrow our choices of animal products during the Elimination Phase because these foods are high on the food chain and contain persistent toxins that stress our immune systems (see chapter 8). They provide concentrated amounts of protein that, in excess, burden our kidneys, bones, and liver (see chapter 16.) Animal products contain cholesterol that, in excess, alters how we process important essential fats (see chapter 6). To avoid these problems and the inflammation they may cause, we restrict ourselves to only certain species of wild fish, some shellfish, skinless chicken or turkey, eggs, and lean cuts of grass-fed lamb.

---

[11] As its name shows, much of the marketing force behind rapeseed oil as a food came from Canada. Canola is short for CANadian low OLeic Acid.

[12] Of course, these days almost all processed and pre-prepared foods contain canola oil so, even if the percentage of erucic acid in the oil is low, we may in fact be ingesting quite a bit overall. It does not appear that the government considered the large amount of canola oil that people would be eating in its evaluation of the healthfulness of canola.

Many other lean animal products come back as daily food choices after the Elimination and Testing Phases. Even the fattier cuts find a place in the eating plan. Eliminating most animal products for a brief period allows us to consciously and individually evaluate how best to incorporate them after the Elimination Phase.

8. ELIMINATE CHEMICALS AND HEAVILY PROCESSED FOODS

We eliminate all chemicals and heavily processed foods: Additives, flavorings, artificial colors, artificial fats, hydrogenated fats, refined grains, modified starches, preservatives, and all non-food ingredients are off-limits. The goal is to eat only real, whole foods. Essentially, the rule is: *If ingredients on the label did not at one time walk, crawl, fly, swim, or grow, or if the ingredients spent any significant time in a laboratory or chemical factory, we do not eat them.* By following this rule, we only eat real food. Another way to implement this rule: Avoid any food that contains an ingredient that you cannot pronounce or cannot explain in detail what it is, how it came into being, and how and *why* it ended up in a food you intend to eat.

The best that can be said for artificial ingredients is that they might not harm us. No one suggests that they are good for us, and no health claims are made for them. On this plan, we eat foods that are good for us, and avoid anything that supposedly does not harm us, but has not been established to be good for us. In fact, many of these "harmless" chemicals deplete our bodies of needed nutrients. Some are outright toxic and generate significant amounts of inflammation.

Another reason to avoid chemicals is that our safety testing systems are inadequate, which means we should not rely on claims that they are safe. A case in point: The most rigorous safety testing is done on prescription drugs before they are approved and brought to market. Millions of dollars and many years are spent establishing the safety and efficacy of a prescription drug going through the approval process. Nonetheless, in a given ten-year period, half of the drugs approved were pulled from the market either for relabeling to provide additional safety data or were removed entirely.

The testing of other chemicals is not as rigorous. Since the early 1900s, more than 80,000 new chemicals have been developed. Most were simply "grandfathered" into our system, approved merely because they were in use when the first safety regulations were enacted. None were tested as rigorously as the prescription drugs. We simply do not have a good basis for concluding that the chemicals added to processed foods are safe and we have many indications that they are not.

None of these chemicals or heavily processed foods are in any way necessary to us; at best they do not harm us. We choose to avoid them entirely.

9. Eliminate non-organic soy and soy products

We eliminate all non-organic soy and soy products (soy milk, tofu, tempeh, etc.) because almost all conventional soy is grown from genetically modified (GM) seeds. People have very different opinions on the benefits or detriments of GM foods. Before you can make a conscious, informed choice about whether to include them in your diet, you need to understand the potential problems they may pose. Until you at the very least have reviewed the chapter on genetic modification (see chapter 20), you should only eat certified organic soy foods. Certified organic foods may not contain genetically modified ingredients; other soy usually is GM but is not labeled as such.

10. Eliminate refined grains

Grains are refined by removing the dark fibrous husks from the grain, turning whole wheat into white flour and turning brown rice into white. Refining removes and discards fiber needed to maintain the health of our intestinal tract (see chapter 5). Nutrients and vitamins are lost, and refining often involves bleaching and other chemical treatments that further reduce the food value of these foods. By the time we eat white rice, rice flour, white flour, and other refined grains, what once was a complex, healthy food has been reduced to long chains of simple sugars. Refined grains raise our blood sugar levels quickly, grow the wrong intestinal microbes, and supply empty calories that generate oxidative stress, while providing little-to-no nutrients to our body. Refined grains are as inflammatory as concentrated sweeteners and must be avoided during the Elimination Phase.

11. ELIMINATE ALCOHOLIC BEVERAGES

We eliminate all alcohol for five weeks. Then we bring it back but in a more thoughtful way that will be less damaging to us.

Wine, especially red wine, has a reputation of being heart healthy. It contains the antioxidant resveratrol and drinking relaxes the mind. The first glass of wine relaxes tension in our blood vessels which is good for the heart. However, the second glass of wine may begin to constrict the blood vessels, reducing any heart benefit. Any amount of alcohol burdens the liver and disrupts sleep. Recently, even the heart benefits of the first glass of wine have been put into question. Alcohol may not be good for us at all. One recent study found that drinking the equivalent of four to six glasses of wine a week could trigger atrial fibrillation (a heart arrhythmia). Alcohol is toxic to fetuses and any amount of alcohol may cause fetal alcohol syndrome. Alcohol consumption correlates with an increase in cancer incidence, albeit slight.[13] Alcohol also depletes our stores of magnesium (see chapter 12).

Alcohol's side effects show that, despite antioxidants such as resveratrol in wine, alcohol causes damage. Many people struggle with the elimination of alcohol. It is, after all, an addictive substance. Be strict about following this rule during the Elimination Phase so you can confirm that you do not need alcohol. You will also benefit from evaluating how alcohol affects how you feel during the day and how you sleep at night. Finally, remember that beer contains both alcohol and wheat. If you drink beer during the Elimination Phase you are shooting yourself in both feet, so to speak.

12. ELIMINATE JUICES, SMOOTHIES, AND "NOT-MILKS"

On this plan, we eat our food; we do not drink it. All juices, juice drinks (vegetable or fruit), food drinks (glasses of almond, rice,

---

[13] There is some evidence that alcohol does not increase the incidence of prostate cancer but rather clear evidence that it increases breast cancer risk. Because of similarities between the two types of cancer, some question the data that alcohol does not have an adverse effect on prostate cancer. The jury is still out on the question.

or other "not milks"), smoothies, and sodas are eliminated. Our beverages are water, mineral water, coffee, tea, and herb teas. You may "whiten" coffee or tea with small amounts of unsweetened non-dairy milks but *only* at meals and snacks. You may add *small* amounts of non-dairy milks to berries or grains. But be careful. Make sure the not-milks do not contain added sugar or canola oil, and count them as grain or protein depending on what they are made from (For example, almond milk is a protein while rice milk is a grain, so you would not have rice milk at breakfast.)

Juices

We do not drink juice because juice raises blood sugar levels much more quickly than whole fruit. As a result, juice is harder on the body. Juicing usually removes the fruit's fiber so each glass of juice contains only the sweet part of the fruit or vegetable. The concentrated sugars—without the fruit or vegetable fiber—starve the beneficial flora and feed the sugar-loving bacteria species in our intestinal tract. This negative effect on our intestinal flora triggers an inflammatory response (see chapter 5).

Juice is undesirable even when a Vitamix or other high-quality juicer incorporates the fiber. Juice with fiber is superior to juice without fiber from the perspective of our intestinal flora, but any juice tempts us to consume more fruit or sweet vegetables than we usually would. We can easily turn a pound of carrots into a glass of juice and drink it as a snack. We most likely would not snack on a pound of carrots. We can easily turn four oranges into juice but are much less likely to eat four whole oranges.

Part of our journey toward health requires us to enter into an honest and respectful communication with our bodies. How much of a fruit does our body care to eat? The answer is found in the amount of whole fruit we would eat, not in how much juice can slide down our throat before our stomach has a chance to speak to the issue. Respecting our body's messages about how much to eat allows us to eat as much as we want, without portion or calorie control. We lose this ability when we drink our food.

Further, the amount of fruit and sweet vegetables we consume is important beyond simply the amount we might eat. Fruits and sweet vegetables contain the fruit sugar fructose. Fructose does not significantly raise our glucose levels but has profound effects on our body. Historically, the human got relatively small amounts of sugars from fruits and sweet vegetables. Most of those foods contain some, but not too much, glucose and fructose along with lots of fiber and other nutrients. Historically, the overall amount of fructose in the diet was low. However, today, North Americans eat about 150 pounds of sugar a year each. About one-third (50 pounds) is in the form of high-fructose corn syrup and about 60 pounds in the form of pure fructose.

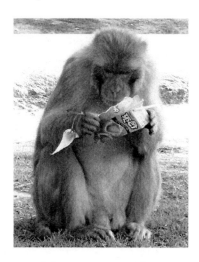

Juices are tempting.

Why are we eating so much fructose in addition to the excessive amount of fructose we get from plain old table sugar? It turns out that fructose is the sweetest of all naturally occurring sugars and synergistically increases sweetness when combined with other sweeteners, both natural and artificial. On its own, fructose is 73 percent sweeter than refined sugar. It is also cheaper than refined sugar. Fructose is increasingly added to our foods to increase profits by engaging our sweet tooth.

Fructose is metabolized by the liver and, although it has little effect on blood sugar levels, it tends to raise blood cholesterol, LDL (the "bad" form of cholesterol), triglycerides, cortisol, and uric acid levels. Excess fructose is bad for heart health. Fructose is associated with gout because of its effect on uric acid. A fructose-rich diet makes our platelets more prone to form clots. It also raises blood pressure. While both glucose and fructose can cause weight gain, fructose increases abdominal fat. Animals on a high-fructose diet rapidly developed fatty livers, much as alcoholics do. Fructose negatively affects hormones involved in appetite control. One study showed that drinking orange juice instead of eating the fruit led to an 18% increased incidence of diabetes over time.

Because fructose is not easily absorbed in the intestines, excess fructose ends up being fermented by the colon flora. This often causes bloating, diarrhea or constipation, flatulence, and pain. Thus, fructose can trigger or aggravate many digestive disorders. Overall, our bodies simply are not designed to handle juices or large amounts of fruit.

To be healthy, we need to drastically reduce fructose in our diet. One of the best ways to begin is to eliminate juices. We should remove them from our children's diets as well. According to the American Pediatric Association, fruit juices are inappropriate for infants and eating fruit is much better than juice for children of all ages. To protect our children's health, we need to teach them to eat fruit and drink water when they are thirsty.

Most people should continue eating fresh fruits. They are rich in fiber, minerals, antioxidants, and vitamins, and they are extremely satisfying. But if you are experiencing bloating, flatulence, diarrhea, constipation, and/or are plateauing on the plan (see chapter 23), you should try to eat less fruit or switch to low-fructose fruits such as berries. You may be ultra-sensitive to fructose, even in small amounts.

Smoothies

We chew to ensure proper digestion of the foods we eat. As we chew, we set in motion a reflex release of digestive enzymes. Our salivary enzymes mix with the food and begin to digest carbohydrates. We secrete stomach acid needed to break down proteins. Other enzymes and bile are released to digest fats. As we chew, we let our brain know what we are eating so that proper amounts of hormones, such as insulin, are released to maintain our blood sugar. This feedback also affects hormones such as grehlin, that influence how full we feel after a meal. There is evidence that chewing triggers satiety signals that liquid foods do not. Although the blender does the job of grinding up the food as well—sometimes even better—than chewing does, it cannot cause us to secrete needed digestive enzymes or affect the amount of grehlin or other metabolic hormones we secrete.

Most smoothies are made from healthy foods. We often blend yoghurt and milk (dairy, rice or nut milks), berries, bananas, and other fruits. Sometimes we include vegetables that either taste sweet (carrots for instance) or whose taste is lost in the sweetness of the fruit mixture. Sometimes we add protein powder, flax seed, wheatgrass juice, and other "nutrients." The smoothie tastes sweet and we drink it quickly. The smoothie spends just enough time in the mouth for our body to register that we are "eating" something sweet. The brain responds by signaling the pancreas to secrete insulin in preparation for a rise in blood sugar. Then, we dump fats and proteins into the stomach before we have signaled the body to release stomach acid and other digestive enzymes. Our digestion must now play catch-up and we are setting the stage for digestive issues: Poorly digested food may allow different strains of microbes to come into dominance. The ensuing change in intestinal flora may inflame the intestinal lining and predispose us to food sensitivities. Our ancestors chewed and ate their food. Smoothies and juices were not available. Our digestive tract is designed to fit our historical diet, and we should eat accordingly.

We are often proud of our smoothies because they are so rich in nutrients. In fact, most of us would not eat all of the foods in the smoothie if we had to eat them separately in one meal with a fork or spoon, especially for breakfast. There is often more fruit than we might eat if we had to peel and chew them, and certainly more fructose than our bodies might want. The components of the smoothie often do not "go well" together: We would not have a cup of soy yoghurt with a sliced banana, a pear, a cup of berries, and a glass of almond milk for breakfast—let alone with a plate of raw kale, protein powder, and a half pound of carrots on the side. We are not trusting our bodies to choose the nutritious foods that we actually need to eat.

Soups are very different from smoothies. Most soups have a savory taste; they are not simply sweet. Many soups are chunky and require some chewing. And we eat soups more slowly with a spoon. This allows the brain and the digestive tract to respond appropriately to what we are eating. We have time to recognize when we have had enough of the soup. In contrast, the sweetness of the smoothie often entices the person to drink the same sweet blend day after day. We seldom eat the same soup days running, and consequently eat a greater variety of foods over time. This helps us get that variety of antioxidants our bodies need (see chapter 7).

Unless you cannot chew, have an ailment that limits how much you can eat, or requires you to eat immense amounts, you should not drink your food. If you absolutely will not give up your smoothies, make sure that they are not sweet treats. Make sure you are not overeating fruit or high-glycemic vegetables and getting too much fructose. Do not cover up the taste of the vegetables you may be adding with fruit and definitely do not add fiberless or sweetened juices to the smoothie. Make sure that the smoothie is proportionate if adding yoghurt or milk of any type. Then sit down and eat your smoothie with a spoon the way you would a soup.

Not-Milks

"Not-milks" made from coconuts, other nuts or grains remove the fiber and, if used as drinks, deliver complex food components too quickly exactly the way most juices do. It is fine to use small amounts of these milks to flavor coffee, soups, and stews, but we should not drink them by the glass nor should we use them by the cupful to make "pseudosweets" (seemingly healthier sweet treats).

13. Eliminate dried fruit

During the Elimination and Testing Phases, we eliminate all dried fruit, including dates. Dried vegetables and dried mushrooms are permitted, but only in cooking.

Dried fruit is added back after the Testing Phase but poses many of the same problems as fruit juice: It is all too easy to eat too much dried fruit, with its concentrated sweet taste and lack of fluid (water), before we feel full. Consider, for example, a fresh mango. Mangoes are luscious, sweet fruits, but they are a bit difficult and messy to cut open. Because of the work and time involved, we are likely to eat one or, at most, two mangoes in any sitting. On the other hand, if we have a bowl of dried, sweet mangoes available, we easily eat many, many mangoes. The result is too much fructose and the resultant inflammation.

Dried fruit can also renew sugar cravings. The concentrated sweet taste pleases our brain, and makes our fruits and vegetables taste less sweet in comparison. Soon, we are craving "real" sweets.

An anecdote:

My friend and I were shopping at Costco. When she placed a giant tub of dates in the cart, I told her not to buy it. "Don't worry," she said, "I only have one—or at most two a day—as dessert and I think that's fine." Four days later, I went to visit her. Her tub of dates was half empty and she was complaining that all of a sudden she was having cravings for sweets that she had not had for a long time. While dried fruit comes back after the Testing Phase, I personally only use it in cooking and avoid keeping it in the house. I even avoid trail mixes with dried fruit in them. Instead, I take apples and a knife, or tangerines and nuts, when I head off on a hike.

---

14. Eliminate any likely trigger foods

Each of us is unique and some of us have more, or different, food sensitivities than others. If you have been told (or suspect) you might be sensitive to eggs, to members of the nightshade family (eggplant, tomatoes, potatoes, and peppers), to tree nuts, to citrus, or any other food, do not eat that food.

If you have a suspected food sensitivity (as opposed to a true food allergy), you may test how you respond to that food when we add foods back in the Testing Phase. But avoid eating any suspect food until then. When we eat a food we are sensitive to, the body will react with inflammation and we will not experience the benefits of quieting inflammation.

CHAPTER FIVE

Tending Our Ecosystem

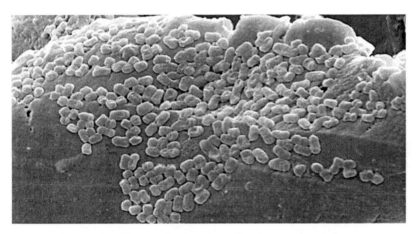

Tens of trillions of microbes live in our intestines.
Together we form a walking ecosystem.

An incredible number of microbes live in our intestinal tract: This long tube that meanders through the middle of our body is populated with somewhere between 10 and 100 trillion microbes. In fact, there are ten times more microbes in that tube than there are cells in our entire body!

These microbes, referred to as our intestinal flora are of many different types and an estimated 1,000 different microbial strains are present there. Most of these microbes are bacteria, but we also host fungi (or yeast) and some protozoa. Some are friends; some are foes. We know quite a bit about the very troublesome species, we have some knowledge about the more dominant species (the beneficial flora), but we know very little about the majority of our intestinal microbes. We do not know what purpose they serve.

We do know that in health beneficial microbes dominate and help us function optimally. Together, we form a synergistic, walking ecosystem in which these microbes play an important part. Put another way, when things are going well, most of the tens of trillions of microbes in our intestines are "good guys" that have an immediate, positive effect on our overall health.

Different microbes specialize in metabolizing certain nutrients, such as sugar, fiber, or fat. Those strains best able to quickly consume a food eaten by us (their host) will use the food's energy to multiply, divide, and become the dominant strain. Those less skilled will get enough food to survive but will not thrive. When we choose what to eat, we are choosing which microbes dominate our ecosystem. Microbes are not long-lived so the composition of our intestinal ecosystem constantly changes as our foods and our digestion changes.[1]

---

[1] Digestion also affects the microflora. A person who digests foods poorly will have larger amounts of incompletely broken down food compounds that will often favor different strains than properly digested food might.

THE INTESTINAL BARRIER

While most of the trillions of these microbes are "our friends," it is still important that they—friend or foe—not invade our body proper. It is important that they respect our intestinal boundaries or borders. In this context, understand that—although the digestive tube is in the middle of our body—the interior of the digestive tube is not part of our body. Instead, our intestinal lining, as does our skin, forms a barrier between us and this "inside-outside" world. Our intestinal lining is an important barrier but one that also must be permeable enough to allow nutrients into our body.

OUR IMMUNE SYSTEM TRACKS OUR MICROBES

Our immune system monitors our intestinal barrier carefully to make sure that the delicate balance, designed to keep microbes and undigested food out while admitting needed nutrients, is properly maintained. The immune system tracks which microbes are dominant and promptly responds with a strong inflammatory response when the wrong microbes are present in too great a number.

Dendrites are immune cells that monitor what is going on in our bodies. In many respects they are the commanding officers of the immune system. Depending on what they find, dendrites will set in motion an inflammatory response or they will quiet ongoing inflammation. They monitor the microbial balance in the intestinal tract with particular care in order to fend off a rise in disease-causing microbes.

To get an idea of how quickly the immune system responds to changes in the flora, think back to a time when you (or some-one else) had food poisoning. A food carried disease-causing bacteria into the intestinal tract. They promptly began multiplying and secreting toxic compounds. The immune system immediately mounted an inflammatory response and flooded the body with cytokines to attract immune cells to the intestinal tract. This inflammatory response caused vomiting and diarrhea (to flush the microbes out of the system) and at the same time caused symptoms such as muscle aches and headaches. In contrast, no such reaction follows when we eat well and grow beneficial microbes. Under those circumstances, things remain happily quiet on the intestinal front.

THE BENEFICIAL MICROBES

We have a long and mutually beneficial relationship with a wide variety of microbes simply because they thrive on foods that historically have been a large part of our diet. They are beneficial because they do good things for us in exchange for the food we provide them, such as:

1. The beneficial strains break down food compounds that we cannot digest on our own. They convert those compounds into energy and excrete byproducts that we absorb and use. One such byproduct is butyric acid/butyrate that appears to prevent the growth of colon polyps. Colon polyps are dangerous because of their ability to turn cancerous and cause colon cancer. These byproducts are also absorbed and bind to cells throughout our body where they enhance our innate ability to prevent cancers from forming. When the immune system comes across a malfunctioning cell, it sends that cell a suicide command, and the cell explodes itself (apoptosis). Precancerous cells tend to ignore suicide commands and continue growing. However, when compounds such as butyrate bind to the precancerous cell, the cell becomes more willing to obey the suicide command. In turn this helps us avoid cancer. These microbial byproducts also shut down the cells' production of a protein that causes inflammation, another precursor to cancer.

2. The beneficial strains produce compounds that shift the pH of our intestinal tract. This improved pH helps us to better absorb important minerals, such as calcium, magnesium, iron, etc. and helps us maintain a healthier intestinal lining.[2] A healthy intestinal lining aids the proper absorption of nutrients and prevents incompletely digested food molecules from crossing the intestinal boundary into the body. Barring entry of larger food molecules into the body proper helps prevent food allergies, food sensitivities, and food intolerances.

---

[2] pH is a measurement of acidity/alkalinity.

3. The beneficial strains produce a form of vitamin K that serves important functions in our body. Vitamin K is necessary for circulatory/heart health and bone health. Too little vitamin K manifests as bleeding and bruising and may lead to liver or gallbladder disease.[3]

4. Our immune system remains calm and does not set in motion an inflammatory response when the beneficial microbes are dominant in our intestinal tract, because we need these microbes to stay healthy. Unlike pathogens, the immune system does not feel threatened by beneficial strains unless the microbes actually cross the intestinal barrier and begin to invade our body proper.

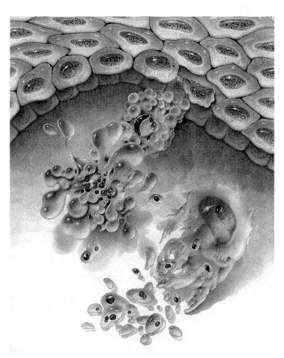

A "wayward" cell following a suicide order
and exploding itself.

---

[3] Diet's effect on blood clotting is particularly important for those taking a blood thinner, such as warfarin. As diet changes, the dose may need to be adjusted. This is one reason why it is important to consult with your health care provider before making dietary changes.

FEEDING OUR FRIENDS

We developed a symbiotic relationship with our beneficials because these microbes thrive on foods that traditionally formed our primary diet, foods rich in fiber, mucilaginous compounds, and complex sugars. First and foremost, these microbes thrive on fiber. We cannot break down fiber ourselves. Instead, we rely on these beneficial microbes in our intestines to digest any fiber we eat. When they metabolize that fiber, they excrete compounds that are useful to us. The fiber in our diet both feeds our good microbes and also helps us maintain an intestinal environment that favors both the good microbes and us. Thus, fiber is an important element of a healthy diet.

Most of us do not provide enough fiber to our good microbes. According to the American Dietetic Association, the average American only gets about 14 to 15 grams of fiber a day. That is about half of the recommended amount of fiber (20 to 35 grams per day), and that recommendation is likely the very least we should get, not the optimum amount of fiber for our bodies.

Beneficial microbes also thrive on complex polysaccharides. Polysaccharides are large, branched sugar chains. These sugars are called complex because their structure is much more intricate than the simple sugars found in white table sugar, honey, or maple syrup. Various types of these important branched sugars are found in mushrooms—from the common little button mushrooms found in the supermarket to the more exotic wild edible mushrooms to the inedible mushrooms used in traditional Asian medicine.

In Japan, one of the many polysaccharides in the turkey tails mushroom (*Trametes versicolor*) has been isolated and is administered as part of conventional treatment of many different types of cancer. Patients take this complex sugar before and after cancer surgery, as well as before and during chemotherapy and radiation treatments. Research shows that this compound prevents conventional cancer treatments from suppressing the patient's immune system but does not interfere with effectiveness of those cancer treatments. This polysaccharide works in part through its effect on the intestinal flora and inflammation.

Another Japanese study showed that people eating at least three ounces of cooked mushrooms a day had a 64 percent lower incidence of cancer compared to people not eating mushrooms. This benefit is probably caused in part because microbial byproducts enhance our innate ability to fight cancer, perhaps by making precancerous cells more sensitive to suicide commands. These studies underscore that eating more mushrooms will both feed our beneficial intestinal flora and support our health.

Another complex sugar, inulin, is found in some root vegetables such as burdock and Jerusalem artichokes (sunchokes). Studies show that people with Crohn's disease, an inflammatory intestinal disorder, appear to have too few of the species *Faecalibacterium prausnitzii* in their intestinal tract. Eating foods rich in inulin increases the number of these bacteria which in turn may have a beneficial effect in Crohn's disease and possibly other digestive ailments.[4]

Vegetables, fruits, whole grains, nuts, and legumes are all rich in fiber and often rich in complex sugars as well. Mushrooms, seaweeds, and many foods common in traditional cuisines provide both fiber and other interesting complex sugars. These foods include daikon, lotus root, okra, cactus pads (or nopales), jicama, bamboo shoots, and water chestnuts. Borrow ethnic cookbooks from the library or look for recipes online that use these vegetables so you can begin to incorporate them into your diet. When eating out, explore dishes with unfamiliar ingredients. For instance, many Mexican restaurants have nopales dishes and Asian restaurants typically have many dishes that include seaweeds, lotus root, burdock, and daikon. This may allow additional strains of good microbes to flourish and benefit you.

---

[4] Inulin is available as a supplement but remember, it is always better to get nourishment from your food, rather than from an isolated compound. Real food contains many compounds that enhance each other's actions. Supplements should be used just as their name implies: They should supplement our diet; they should not be used as a substitute for real foods.

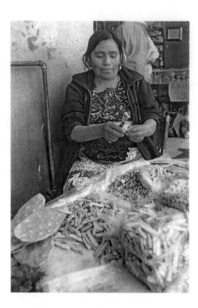

Cactus pads feed our
beneficial microbes.

TROUBLESOME MICROBES

Foods that feed our beneficial microbes are no longer the dominant foods in our diet. In fact, they are relatively rare. Unfortunately, the microbes that are most efficient at metabolizing our typical Western diet are the more troublesome microbes. They are troublesome because they do not benefit our health:

1. They do not produce compounds that prevent polyps, nor do they activate our innate cancer-fighting capacities.

2. The byproducts these microbes excrete change the pH of the intestinal tract but in the wrong direction. This change makes us less able to absorb important minerals. This pH change also tends to inflame our intestinal lining and makes that barrier more porous. In turn, this increases the likelihood that larger food molecules will make it across the lining and into our body proper where they may trigger food allergies and sensitivities. The inflamed membrane also makes us more prone to digestive disorders.

3. These microbes do not produce bacterial vitamin K and do not help us maintain bone and circulatory health.

Our immune system becomes concerned when troublesome microbes start crowding out the beneficial strains. It responds as if the increased numbers of the "wrong" bacteria signal that an invasion may be underway. Immune cells begin to secrete inflammatory cytokines to attract additional immune cells so the body is prepared to fight off any such invasion.

The cytokines secreted when troublesome microbes crowd out the beneficials are the same cytokines that the immune system secretes in response to a cold or flu virus. Depending on the resulting imbalance of different cytokines, this increase in inflammatory cytokines may trigger any number of symptoms, for example fatigue, headaches, joint aches, muscle aches, sinus congestion, and digestive problems to name a few. This is why feeding and growing the wrong flora triggers inflammation. This is why choosing to grow healthy intestinal flora can have a profound impact on your health and well-being. It is also why a change in eating patterns can relieve one person of headaches while relieving another of joint pain.

FEEDING THE TROUBLE MAKERS

The Western diet is rich in simple sugars, refined grains, juices, and animal products. Many of the troublesome microbes are specialists at metabolizing simple sugars and refined grains. (Refined grains are essentially long chains of simple sugars that many strains of bacteria process quickly.) Sugar-loving microbes also thrive on most juices because juicing usually removes the fruit's fiber and concentrates its fruit sugars. In addition, we often drink more food than we might eat: Most people would not eat a pound of carrots as a snack but might easily drink that amount of carrot juice.

Other strains of microbes specialize in the fats and proteins in animal products (meat, dairy, eggs, and fish). Animal products contain neither fiber nor complex sugars. They do not provide much food for our beneficial friends. When our diet is too high in sugars and animals fats and too low in fiber and complex sugars, the wrong flora dominate and we become inflamed.

CHANGING OUR INTERNAL ECOSYSTEM

The modern industrialized diet has shifted away from traditional foods rich in fibers and polysaccharides. This dietary change is a common cause of inflammation. Fortunately, digestive microbes are short-lived so we can quickly shift our intestinal balance to what it should be.[5] As the intestinal environment improves, we begin to heal the intestinal lining. This healing takes longer but, over time, a diet that feeds the right flora can help us overcome food sensitivities, reduce seasonal allergies and asthma, and help heal various disorders, such as irritable bowel syndrome.

In studies, people with diets high in miso, seaweed, apples, and naturally brewed soy sauce have fewer allergic symptoms. Those foods all contain complex sugars. A probiotic supplement of good bacteria (see below) boosted the ability of long-distance runners to cope with colds and flu, and cut their respiratory infections by half. These studies combine to show how maintaining healthy intestinal flora directly affects immune system function and our health.

On the TQI Diet, the proportionate meal provides a simple, fail-proof way to maintain a healthy population of the good flora. When we eat proportionately, every meal provides fiber and complex sugars for our beneficial flora to eat. Basically, we feed our beneficials at every meal and snack. At least half of breakfast consists of fruits and vegetables rich in fiber. All other meals and snacks provide twice as much food for the "good guys." This simple method ensures that the beneficial microbes are dominant in our intestines. If, in addition, we avoid sugars, processed foods, and chemicals while limiting our intake of animal products, we guarantee that our beneficial flora will thrive.

---

[5]   Bacteria are short-lived but they reproduce quickly, producing voluminous numbers of offspring. They fill the intestinal space and crowd out other species. When their favored food sources are depleted, their reproductive rate slows. They are able to metabolize other food compounds but not as efficiently as other strains. Other species may then become dominant. There can be rapid shifts in the dominant species but none of our many strains die out completely. They simply remain in semi-hibernation waiting for the right moment (or food) to bloom again.

Fermented Foods and Probiotics

We can also help maintain a rich mixture of beneficial strains in our digestive tract by eating fermented foods. These foods carry—and feed—interesting microbes that support intestinal health. Each ethnic culture has fermented foods, such as sauerkraut and kimchee, and we should definitely work on including some of these foods in our diet. Yoghurt is also a fermented food. However, because it is a fiberless animal product, it does not do as good a job for us as kimchee or sauerkraut. Yoghurt contains good bacteria but it is also an animal product that encourages the growth of bacterial strains that ultimately will tend to hinder somewhat the absorption of minerals. Thus studies show that people absorb more calcium from kale than they do from milk, most likely a result of the differing effects dairy and kale have on the growth of different microbes. The negative effect of yoghurt will, of course, be greater if the yoghurt is sweetened (which most are) or is poorly made and does not contain live bacteria.

People also try to maintain a healthy intestinal flora by taking probiotic supplements. Probiotics provide billions of, at most, a handful of strains of beneficial microbes. They can certainly be useful during travel to countries where unfamiliar strains of bacteria activate the immune system resulting in cases of traveler's diarrhea. Probiotics also help maintain some semblance of intestinal health during a course of antibiotics.

Nonetheless, probiotics are vastly inferior to growing our own strains by eating the right foods. Remember, we have a multitude of beneficial strains of bacteria waiting for the right food. Probiotics provide only a few strains of bacteria, whereas the right foods will feed hundreds of different strains of microbes. In addition, it is becoming increasingly difficult to ascertain whether the strains used in yoghurts and capsules are patented, genetically engineered bacteria that we may not want to have settle into our intestinal tracts. The wiser course is to eat the "prebiotic" foods described above that will grow a variety of beneficial strains and, again, reserve well chosen supplements for special circumstances where you need an extra boost.

CHAPTER SUMMARY

One of the reasons why the TQI Diet works so fast and so well is because it provides significant support to our microbial ecosystem and we can quickly improve our flora. As the balance of good flora improves, inflammation subsides. As inflammation subsides, our condition improves. People usually notice signs of improvement in the first few days on the TQI Diet. These rapid changes are also one of the reasons why it is important to adhere closely to the recommended foods during the Elimination Phase. When we make exceptions, we disturb the balance of microbes in the intestinal flora and inflammation increases immediately.

CHAPTER SIX
Essential Fats in Balance

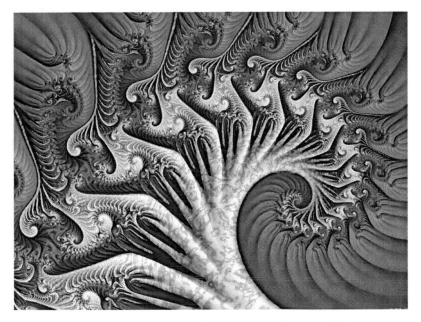

A fractal of broccoli, a plant source of essential fats.

Fats are critical to good health because every single cell in our body needs fats to function. Fats make up the wall, or membrane, around each cell. Inside the cell, we have various organelles that keep the cell functioning, and each organelle is surrounded by its own fatty membrane. Finally, the cell's nucleus where our DNA is stored has a membrane, also composed of fats.

Each membrane needs a high degree of fluidity to make it possible for molecules to move in and out of the cell, organelle, or nucleus. Membranes also need a certain amount of rigidity so we do not ooze away. The body makes from scratch most of the many different fats we need for these membranes. We do not need to eat fats in order to make them. However, there are two groups of fats our body cannot make: Omega-6 fats and omega-3 fats. These are called essential fats because we cannot live without them. We must get them in our daily diet and they are essential to life.

Plants have the unique ability to make both omega-6 and omega-3 fats. They can also convert omega-6s into -3s and omega-3s into -6s, a skill humans and animals do not have. Instead, we must get both types of essential fats from our diet. Plants make omega-3s primarily for use in the membranes that surround the plants' chloroplasts, which is where plants harvest sunshine and convert it into plant matter. The chloroplasts (and thus the omega-3 fats) are concentrated in the above ground parts of plants, usually in the parts that have a green color.

Sunshine is a powerful energy source that provides great benefits but one that also can cause damage. We need sunshine to activate vitamin D (a hormone critical to our health and survival) but too much solar radiation will damage our skin and cause skin cancers. Similarly, plants need sunshine to grow but excess solar radiation can damage their tissue and DNA. Plants use omega-3 fats to protect against the potentially damaging effects of sunshine.

Omega-3 fats are highly reactive. They interact with excess solar radiation and prevent it from damaging the plant. That is why plants concentrate omega-3 fats in their chloroplasts where they process solar energy. The reactivity of omega-3 fats, however, comes with fragility. If left sitting around, they will react with air molecules and become rancid. Omega-3 fats get rancid much more quickly than other types of fats and once rancid, they provide no protection and actually cause damage.

In contrast, omega-6s are very stable fats, much less reactive, and much less prone to get rancid. Plant seeds may sit around for months, years, or even many decades before they germinate. Therefore, plants make and store fats for future seedlings in the form of omega-6s. The stability of omega-6 fats ensures that plant seeds contain a non-rancid store of energy for growth.

When the seed germinates and the seedling begins to grow, the seedling converts the more stable omega-6s back into omega-3s and incorporates them in its chloroplasts. The omega-3 fats then, as described above, protect the seedling from excess solar radiation as it grows.

We borrow and use omega-3s and omega-6s in much the same way as plants do. We incorporate the omega-3 fats in our membranes to protect our cells and our DNA from damage. Omega-3 fats are very important in brain and nerve functioning, eyesight, and glucose metabolism. They also directly affect our immune system, causing it to produce fewer inflammatory cytokines. In our bodies, omega-3 fats are anti-inflammatory.

We use omega-6 fats in cell membranes because they are stable. Our body uses omega-6s in fat storage, to maintain a degree of cell wall rigidity, and for blood clotting. Omega-6s also have a direct effect on our immune system. They increase the production of inflammatory cytokines and support the body's inflammatory response. In our bodies, omega-6 fats are inflammatory.

An appropriate ratio of omega-6s and -3s is critical to our health because they affect the inflammatory response. We need both fats in balance because an imbalance will exaggerate either the inflammatory or anti-inflammatory effect of the fat present in excess. Ideally, our ratio of omega-6 to omega-3 (omega-6:3) fats should be 1.5:1 or just slightly more omega-6 than omega-3.[1]

Unfortunately, our modern diet distorts the ratio of these two fats to our detriment. In most Americans, the ratio of omega-6:3 is heavily weighted toward the inflammatory omega-6 fats. Many of us have a ratio of 20:1 with vegetarians and vegans often having the most distorted ratios. With a ratio of 20:1, our immune system is receiving some twenty signals to produce inflammatory cytokines to each signal to quiet inflammation.

We are inflamed because our diet does not contain enough omega-3 (or anti-inflammatory) fats and contains far too many omega-6 (inflammatory) fats. To change this inflammatory imbalance, we must change what we eat.

WHAT WE EAT DETERMINES OUR OMEGA FAT RATIO
FOODS WE SHOULD EAT

Historically, the human diet was rich in leafy greens and green vegetables, the parts of plants where the chloroplasts and the omega-3 fats are concentrated. Today, when we eat vegetables at all, we favor roots (carrots, beets, potatoes) or fruits (tomatoes, peppers, cucumbers). Most of the vegetables we eat are not rich in chloroplasts, and usually do not provide omega-3 fats.

The human diet used to be richer in berries rather than the sweeter fruits we favor today. Berries are a good source of omega-3 fats; the wilder the berry, the more omega-3s in the berry. Other fruits do not provide many, if any, omega-3 fats.

Historically, animal products in the human diet came from lean animals that roamed, grazing or browsing on green plants. Land animals that live a natural life eating their intended diet have a good ratio of omega-6:3 fats. Eggs came from wild birds. Eggs from chickens that forage on weeds, seeds, and insects have an omega-6:3 ratio of about 1.5:1—an ideal ratio for us. Fish in the diet were always wild. Wild fish are a rich source of omega-3 fats because their diet consists entirely of green water plants (phytoplankton) or smaller fish that live on phytoplankton.

---

[1] Although it may seem wrong, convention first lists the omega-6 content compared to the omega-3 content. This ratio is given as 6:3 1.5:1. So the first number pertains to omega-6 content, the second to omega-3.

FOODS WE SHOULD EAT LESS OF

Few people today eat a diet rich in green vegetables, wild berries, and animal products from lean animals fed their natural diet. Instead, we eat a great deal of grain, particularly in the form of wheat and processed corn. Grains are seeds and seeds are usually higher in inflammatory omega-6 fats.

We eat wheat at virtually every meal and snack. We eat it as bread, granola, or oatmeal at breakfast. We have sandwiches for lunch, cookies for snacks, and pasta or burgers for dinner. The latter come surrounded by buns and are filled with bread crumbs. We also eat a lot of dried corn products, and corn is another seed higher in omega-6s. Most of our dried corn comes in the form of corn oil presented as vegetable oil but we also get a lot of dried corn from fast food and processed foods. Fast foods, at their core, are corn.[2]

Whatever corn we do not eat ourselves, we feed to our animals, even though most of them need grass or other green plants to be healthy. The grain diet has a dramatic effect on their omega-6:3 ratio. A North Dakota State University study on the nutritional differences between grass-fed and grain-fed bison found that grass-fed bison had omega-6:3 ratios of 4:1, while the grain-fed bison had ratios of 21:1. Some studies found factory-farmed meat to have a ratio as high as 40:1. An average supermarket egg can run 19:1 because the diet of factory-farmed chicken is poor and nearly devoid of omega-3 fats.

We do not eat fish often. When we do, we usually eat farmed fish, often breaded (more wheat) and deep-fat fried.[3] Farmed fish do not live on phytoplankton but instead are usually fed fish pellets, a kibble high in omega-6 fats. Farmed fish consistently are high in omega-6 fats in contrast to wild fish that are a fabulous source of omega-3 fats.

We also often eat processed foods. Processed, prepackaged foods contain manipulated vegetable oils. As they are manipulat-

---

[2] One study found that 469 out of 470 fast-food meals at their core consisted of corn and corn products.

[3] Most restaurants, for instance, serve Atlantic salmon, which is always farmed. And in most parts of the country, all seafood on the menu will be farmed and high in omega-6 fats.

ed or "deodorized," any omega-3 fats in the original vegetable oils are destroyed—sometimes accidentally but more often intentionally—to improve the shelf life of the final products. (Remember, omega-3 fats tend to go rancid quickly.) In addition, plants such as soybeans and rape seed (used to make canola) are often hybridized to produce fewer omega-3 fats, again so foods made from them will not spoil as quickly. Finally, many foods are prepared with high omega-6 fats, such corn, safflower, or sunflower oil.

WHY VEGANS AND VEGETARIANS OFTEN HAVE A POOR RATIO

Today, because of unwise food choices, many of us have a ratio of omega-6:3 as high as 20:1. While vegetables provide omega-3s, most vegans (who exclude all animal products from their diet) often have a worse ratio than omnivores because many vegans primarily eat grains and root vegetables. They do not necessarily favor plant foods high in omega-3s.[4] Vegetarians often have a yet greater imbalance because they add grain-fed dairy and factory-farmed eggs to the vegan-type grain diet but do not eat any wild fish. Both diets can be healthy but only if they contain enough omega-3 fats. Ultimately, we all struggle with an inflammatory imbalance of omega-6:3s because we have moved away from our historical diet that was high in green foods and low in grains.

RESTORING OUR OMEGA-6:3 BALANCE

Symptoms of an imbalance of omega-6:3 are varied and include: Aching, painful joints and muscles; anovulatory menstrual cycles; chest pains; cracked nails; depression; dry hair and skin; dry mucous membranes, tear ducts, mouth, vagina; eczema, psoriasis and other skin conditions; fatigue, malaise, lackluster energy; forgetfulness; frequent colds and sickness; inability to concentrate; hyperactivity; indigestion, gas, bloating; irregular heartbeat; lack of endurance, lack of motivation; and premature skin wrinkling.

In the Elimination Phase, we immediately begin to restore our omega-6:3 balance. First, we eliminate our two favorite grains:

---

[4]   The recipes in most vegan cookbooks are for grain dishes made with wheat or rice with very few recipes rich in leafy green vegetables.

Wheat and dried corn. We also limit the overall amount of grain in the diet by applying the Rule of Proportions to every meal and snack. But we need to do more to overcome our omega-6:3 imbalance. We need to make a dedicated effort to change our diet and:

 Eat more leafy greens (such as lettuce, kale, chard, purslane, spinach, dandelion leaves, nettles, etc.), and more green plants[5] (cabbage, broccoli, etc.) while eating far fewer grains.[6]

 Eat more berries, especially wild berries. All berries are rich in omega-3s, and wild berries have more omega-3s than cultivated berries.

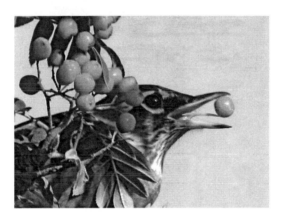

Berries are Rich in Essential Fats

 Eat more walnuts and pumpkin seeds because they have a better omega-6:3 ratio. Or drizzle some walnut or pumpkinseed oil on salads and vegetables.

 Use olive oil as our main oil (it is an omega-9 oil that has a neutral effect on our omega-6:3 ratio). Many sources recommend canola oil because it has a relatively good balance of omega-6:3 fats. On this plan, however, we avoid canola oil because it contains

---

[5] Most of these vegetables will be green in color but some, such as cabbage and cauliflower, may be white, yellow, red, or purple.

[6] While wheat and dried corn are the most common grains in our diet, rice, buckwheat, and other grains also are higher in omega-6 fats.

erucic acid and is being hybridized to provide fewer omega-3 fats. We use other oils for flavor only and do not use large quantities of oils high in omega-6 fats (such as safflower and sunflower oils). We completely eliminate corn oil, another high omega-6 oil.

🍎 Eat ground flax, chia, or hemp seed, or use flax or hemp oil (these seeds are high in omega-3s).

🍎 Eat a variety of *wild*, coldwater fish. Farmed fish are *not* a good source of omega-3s and should not be eaten.

🍎 Eat only lean grass-fed *and* grass-finished animals, or dairy products from such animals, because a grass diet improves the animal's omega-6:3 ratio which in turn will affect our omega-6:3 ratio.

🍎 Eat only eggs and meat from "pastured" chickens eating a natural, healthy diet or eggs from chickens fed omega-3 rich seeds (such as flax).

🍎 Eat proportionately to avoid overeating grains. Favor wild fish and other foods higher in omega-3s over whole grains (such as brown rice) at most meals and snacks.

🍎 Avoid processed foods. Refined carbohydrates (such as white rice and white flour) affect our ability to use essential fats. Metabolizing refined foods actually robs the body's store of nutrients. Without these nutrients, we cannot metabolize fats and cholesterol properly. Cholesterol levels rise, as do our blood sugar levels. High blood sugar inhibits the release of essential fats from storage, resulting in a deficiency even where essential fatty acids are available.

🍎 Avoid supplements that are "complete omegas" or are high in omega-6s. We only need omega-3s from our supplements.

🍎 Limit the amount of saturated animal fats in the diet. A diet rich in bad fats and refined carbohydrates increases the production of cholesterol; this effect is exaggerated if we consume a lot of dietary cholesterol. In excess, saturated animal fats limit the body's ability to use essential fats.

CHAPTER SUMMARY

Maintaining an appropriate balance of omega-6:3 fats is a challenge for most of us: We like our sugars, grains, and animal products. We are often unwilling to pay the higher price for quality animal products. And we are not especially inclined to eat enough green vegetables. It takes a consistent, conscious effort to ensure that our daily food, ideally every meal, includes omega-3 fats. This effort is needed because we cannot quiet inflammation if our omega-6:3 ratio is out of balance.

ALZHEIMER'S DISEASE, AND MULTIPLE SCLEROSIS

Omega-3 fats may slow the development of two brain lesions that are hallmarks of Alzheimer's disease (protein tangles and beta-amyloid). In a study, mice in a control group ate foods with an omega-6:3 ratio of 10:1. They were compared to mice eating food with an omega-6:3 ratio of 1:1. After three months, mice eating a better ratio of omega-6:3 had lower levels of both protein tangles and beta-amyloid.

Other studies strongly suggest that getting enough omega-3 fats may provide a measure of relief for those with multiple sclerosis.

CHAPTER SEVEN

Antioxidants

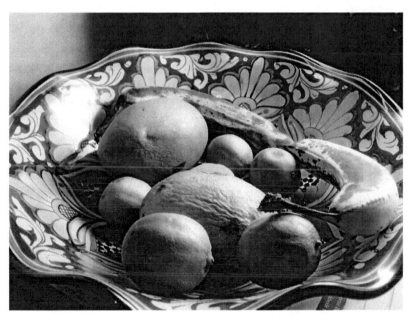

Oxidative stress causes fruit to wrinkle and brown.

Most of us know that antioxidants are good for us. In fact, we periodically buy expensive tropical juices and supplements in the belief that their rich concentrations of antioxidants will provide great health benefits. Nonetheless, most of us do not know why we need antioxidants or even what they are. Simply put, antioxidants are compounds that prevent oxidative stress damage.

WHAT IS OXIDATIVE STRESS?

Oxidative stress occurs at the molecular level. All atoms have specific numbers of electrons circling around their nuclei. These atoms are harmonious (or nonreactive) when a full set of electrons is in orbit. However, if a beam of light passes through the atom, or a highly reactive chemical is in the vicinity, electrons may either be knocked off their orbit or simply stolen away.

Some atoms do not tolerate losing electrons and become free radicals when they do. Free radicals are disharmonious—or reactive—and will grab a replacement electron from wherever they can. Oxygen is the best-known atom of this kind. Free radicals damage other atoms by stealing their electrons. The resulting damage is called oxidative stress.

Oxidative stress creates many different types of damage. It is what causes an unappealing brownish layer to form on the surface of an apple or avocado sliced in half and left out in the open. Oxidative stress is what causes metal tools left out in the weather to rust and crumble. Oxidative stress also damages our bodies. The aging and wrinkling of our skin is another example of oxidative stress damage.

Free radicals are generated every time energy is changed from one form to another, and we create free radicals when we eat and when we exercise. We change the oxygen we breathe into a usable cellular energy form in organelles called mitochondria.

This process generates numerous free radical oxygen molecules that diffuse throughout our cells looking for electrons. These free radicals take electrons from fats in our membranes, from proteins our bodies need to function, and even from our DNA. This free radical action can damage us in a way that adds up to serious problems over time.

How antioxidants prevent oxidative stress damage

The body uses antioxidants to prevent oxidative stress damage. An antioxidant will donate an electron to a free radical oxygen atom that is hunting for a replacement electron. Once the oxygen molecule has the right number of electrons back in orbit, it becomes harmonious again. Of course, this leaves the antioxidant out of balance, without the right number of electrons. If the depleted antioxidant is forced to go too long without a replacement electron, it will eventually become a free radical itself. We prevent this from happening by maintaining a large supply of different antioxidants in our bodies.

We need a wide variety of antioxidants because they essentially play a game of hot potato with each other, with the missing electron being the hot potato. For instance, the antioxidant vitamin C donates an electron to an oxygen free radical. Soon, a different antioxidant, perhaps vitamin E, donates an electron to the depleted Vitamin C, dampening its reactivity. This continues down the line with different types of antioxidants restoring stability to other antioxidants until the potato is cold and the reactivity entirely dampened.[1]

Studies show that we must maintain a variety of different antioxidants to prevent oxidative stress damage. For this variety to be achieved, we must have plant foods in our diet. Plants contain an incredible variety of antioxidants and an optimal diet could provide some 4,000 different antioxidants. These antioxidants

---

[1] This is, of course, a simplified explanation of the forces in effect but nonetheless is reasonably accurate for our purposes. Molecules do not always donate electrons, they share them and this helps dampen—or cool—that hot potato (i.e., the missing electron), ending the chain reaction.

include vitamins (e.g., vitamins C and E), minerals (e.g., selenium), and numerous other antioxidant compounds such as carotenoids from carrots, lycopene from tomatoes, and lutein from bilberries.

One interesting study on the importance of antioxidants looked at the diets of Finnish men. It found that male smokers who ate lots of fruits and vegetables developed less lung cancer than did male non-smokers not eating many fruits and vegetables. The health benefits of eating fruits and vegetables were impressive but in several respects the study was flawed from a scientific point of view. The study relied on people remembering (and being honest about) what they ate; a problem because people are notoriously poor at this. The antioxidant-content of the fruits and vegetables probably was responsible for the significant health benefits seen. But because so many different plant compounds were in play in their foods, no firm conclusions could be drawn about exactly which one protected these men from lung cancer.

To remedy these issues, a prospective study was launched in which one group of men took a placebo pill and a second group took a beta-carotene supplement.[2] At the end of the study, the men taking beta-carotene had a slightly higher incidence of cancer. What happened? Without a rich variety of antioxidants to play the game of hot potato with free radicals, the beta-carotene itself eventually became a free radical and began to damage the body, increasing the incidence of cancer. Other studies found that vitamin C or E provided as a supplement had similar effects. In summary, to prevent oxidative stress damage, we need a variety of antioxidants available to our cells at the moment they are needed and we need to get our antioxidants from our food.[3]

Unfortunately, most of us do not get enough antioxidants to counteract oxidative stress. We instead experience the common symptoms of oxidative stress damage: Fatigue, poor mental function, mood disorders (e.g., depression, anxiety, etc.), poor immune

---

[2]   Beta-carotene is one of the many carotenoids in, for instance, carrots.

[3]   This is not to suggest that supplements are bad for us. Instead, it is a reminder that supplements should be used to supplement a healthy diet and should be chosen carefully by someone knowledgeable about their effects as well as the individual's need for a particular supplement.

function (making us catch virtually every cold that goes around), joint and muscle aches, headaches, and allergies, to name just a few. Unchecked oxidative stress is inflammatory because it damages our cells and organelles. This damage attracts the attention of our immune cells and they will attempt to fix that damage via an inflammatory response. Unfortunately, the immune system cannot remedy the problem and instead generates chronic inflammation. The proportionate meal ensures that we always have a rich variety of antioxidants available to prevent oxidative stress damage.

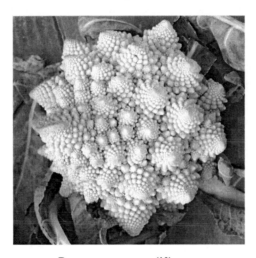

Romanesco cauliflower

ANTIOXIDANTS ARE FOUND IN ALL PLANTS

Antioxidants give plant foods their colors. The glorious shades of purple in eggplant; the greens, yellows, and reds of tomatoes and peppers; the red, orange, yellow, and green of squashes; the white of cauliflower and daikon—all are due to different antioxidants. All are useful and none is better than any other—even if some receive more media coverage than others.[4] We need them in abundance and we need their differences. We absorb antioxidants more easily when we eat foods that have ripened naturally, so it is good to eat seasonally. One of our goals is to eat a variety of plant foods in their season—a good thing because variety also prevents boredom.

---

[4] Examples of antioxidants better covered in the media include vitamin C, resveratrol, lycopene, and beta-carotene.

SOURCES OF OXIDATIVE STRESS

FOOD

Of course, in order to prevent oxidative stress damage, we need to understand what creates free radicals. For most of us, the food we eat is a primary source of oxidative stress. Remember, we generate free radicals every time we transform energy from one form to another, which is exactly what we do when we eat. If we eat a carrot, transforming the plant compounds into calories generates free radicals. The carrot, however, also provides antioxidants that can immediately quiet those free radicals and leave antioxidants to spare. Most of us, however, eat high-calorie food that contains little-to-no antioxidants. Animal products, refined grains, sugars, and empty calories generate massive amounts of free radicals but do not provide antioxidants to prevent oxidative stress damage.

It is also important to understand the time scale that molecules operate on: In the blink of an eye, multitudes of free radicals can be generated that will immediately begin stealing electrons from within our cells. To prevent that damage, we need antioxidants the moment those free radicals are generated, not hours later.[5]

BAD FATS

Bad dietary fats generate large amounts of oxidative stress. We have enzymes that break apart, digest, and build fats. These enzymes basically chomp along fat molecules expecting—and needing—particular bonds at particular places. Our enzymes can handle all of the fats that historically have been part of our diet. But today's industrialized foods supply many fats with entirely new bonds that our enzymes cannot process.

Curiously, the natural, unrefined oils usually have their own section in the grocery store. They are typically bottled in dark glass to reduce oxidation of the oil by light. Aisles away, other shelves are stocked with inexpensive vegetable oils usually sold

---

[5]   When we eat a charbroiled steak or sugary dessert at one meal and then eat our antioxidants at some later meal, the antioxidants may be able to repair the damage done by the earlier meal but will not be able to prevent it. Simply put: If we want to *prevent* oxidative stress damage, we need antioxidants to be part of every meal.

in clear plastic bottles. These latter oils have been refined and deodorized. To deodorize oil, manufacturers heat the oil to between 400 and 500 degrees Fahrenheit. The oils are heated to destroy omega-3 fats because omega-3 fats are reactive and tend to go rancid quickly (hence the need to "deodorize"). By destroying the desirable omega-3 fats, the shelf life of the oil is increased. But in the process, new types of chemical bonds are created, including trans-fat bonds. These chemical bonds are not found in nature. Fat digestion stops when the enzyme encounters a strange bond and the undigested remnant is stored in globs (lipofuscin) in the cell. Massive amounts of oxidative stress are generated as the body tries to deal with these fats. This is one of the reasons why trans-fats are associated with so many health problems.

On this plan, we are free to eat as much good fat (such as oils from avocados and nuts) as our body craves, but we are not to eat any bad fats. If we slip and eat them (usually when we indulge in fast food or prepackaged food), we will need many additional antioxidants to prevent those bad fats from damaging the body and we need to have them with the meal that contains bad fats.

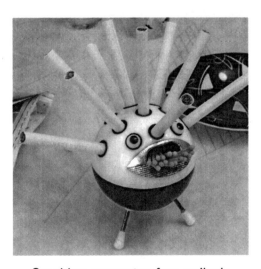

Smoking generates free radicals

SMOKING

Smoking generates free radicals. If you inhale cigarette smoke, you inhale highly reactive chemicals. Those chemical free radicals, unchecked, may steal electrons from the DNA in your lungs, initiating lung cancer. If you smoke, you need great quantities of antioxidants to help your body *attempt* to counter this effect.

ALCOHOL

Drinking alcohol also generates free radicals. Additionally, alcohol places a burden on the liver and can cause fatty liver and cirrhosis. Alcohol is quickly dispersed throughout our body and is toxic to all of our cells. That is why any amount of alcohol is associated with a slightly increased incidence of cancer. In our culture, alcohol is an important relaxant for many, and most people are going to drink alcohol periodically. It "comes back" to the diet after the Elimination and Testing Phases. When it does, we will discuss how we can offset and mitigate some of the oxidative stress that alcohol generates. Essentially, we make sure that we consume antioxidants with any alcohol we drink.

INSUFFICIENT SLEEP

Insufficient sleep increases free radicals. As we sleep, we generate less metabolic waste and give our body time to repair itself. We need this repair time to maintain our overall health. When we do not sleep enough (or do not sleep well), metabolic waste begins to accumulate. Metabolic waste is another term for oxidative stress. Thus, during periods where our work schedule or our stress level limits our sleep, we need to compensate by eating more antioxidants. We also need to be more meticulous about avoiding high-calorie, antioxidant-poor foods.

RADIATION

Any beam or ray that can pass through our body has the potential to knock electrons off their orbits, including cell phone waves, wifi, x-rays, radioactive fallout, and radon, to name a few. Our lives are filled with ever-increasing amounts and new types of radiation and we need to increase our antioxidants to match. A classic example is excess solar radiation. As sun rays hit the skin, they knock electrons off their orbits, creating free radicals. If those free radicals take electrons from our collagen, we suffer premature aging of the skin. If they take the electrons from our DNA, we develop skin cancer. Adding more antioxidants to our diet helps mitigate this damage.

Pollution

Pollution consists of reactive chemicals that enter our body and steal electrons from within our cells. In today's world, it is impossible to avoid all pollution, and we all need extra antioxidants to help lessen the damage those chemicals cause.

Demanding workouts

Strenuous exercise is good for us. However, it does generate significant amounts of free radicals because, as we exercise, we break down stored energy and convert it to burnable energy. As mentioned earlier, converting energy from one form to another generates free radicals. To cope with these additional free radicals, we need to increase our antioxidant intake when we engage in demanding workouts.

Inadequate exercise

At the other end of the spectrum, no—or too little—exercise is damaging to the body. Humans are designed to move and, as we move, we generate compounds critical to our health, especially the health of our liver. So, if because of pain, weight, or time constraints we are not exercising, our levels of free radicals increase. We can help prevent the resulting damage by simply eating more fruits and vegetables and more carefully avoiding empty calories during low activity periods.

Injuries, infections, and seasonal allergies

Injuries, infections, and seasonal allergies generate metabolic waste. We speed healing by increasing our antioxidant intake when we are ill or injured. For instance, health food stores often recommend the food supplement quercetin to quiet symptoms of mild-to-moderate seasonal allergies. Quercetin is an antioxidant found in onions and watermelon. Its positive action in reducing symptoms of seasonal allergies shows how a well-chosen antioxidant, along with a good diet, can prevent the ill effects that otherwise would arise from excess oxidative stress.

Drugs and medications also generate oxidative stress. All pharmaceuticals come with side effects that are in part caused by oxidative stress. If you are taking medications, you may find that an antioxidant-rich diet will help protect you from the side effects of those drugs without in any way negating the beneficial actions the drugs are designed to provide.

A DOZEN WAYS TO REDUCE OXIDATIVE STRESS

1. Avoid foods that provide empty calories. Make it your goal never to eat antioxidant-poor foods alone, always have fruits or vegetables too—the more the better. The proportionate meal ensures this.

2. Avoid charred or charbroiled animal products (e.g., meat, chicken). Charbroiling generates highly reactive compounds called heterocyclic amines that are very harmful. If and when you eat such foods, make sure you have an ample amount of vegetables.

3. Avoid food excesses. We do not need turkeys stuffed with butter-laden, white-bread dressing, wrapped in bacon, and served with gravy made with cream. We do not need platter-sized steaks, and if we eat one, it is important to remember to eat two platter-sized servings of vegetables with that steak to reduce the oxidative stress it generates.

4. Avoid plastic wrappers and bottles that leach bisphenols and other reactive chemicals.

5. Avoid pesticide, herbicide, and fungicide residues on food.

6. Avoid stress to the greatest extent possible; both emotional and physical stress generate free radicals. Eat more carefully when you are under stress.

7. Get sufficient sleep; it is healing to both mind and body. If you are sleep-deprived, compensate by eating more antioxidants and more carefully avoiding inflammatory foods.

8. Eat as many berries as you can, the wilder the better. They contain strong antioxidants and provide significant health benefits.

9.   Eat leafy greens. They provide interesting antioxidants, fiber for your intestinal flora, and omega-3 fats.

10. Use herbs and spices in your cooking. Herbs and spices carry a tremendous amount of antioxidant compounds in very small packages. Take ginger, for instance: A study shows that ginger powder can offset chemotherapy's tendency to cause nausea and vomiting. Turmeric, a related root, has been the subject of thousands of studies. It is a strong antioxidant that appears to relieve joint pain.

And do not disregard the milder European cooking herbs, such as rosemary, thyme, and oregano. In response to market surveys showing that consumers prefer salad dressings without chemical preservatives, manufacturers discovered that adding rosemary to a salad dressing prevents the oil from going rancid. In other words, rosemary quiets the free radicals that would damage the oil which, no doubt, is why humans typically add herbs and spices to dressings: They keep the oil fresh and they will keep our cells fresh as well.

11. Learn to enjoy the bounty. Choosing health requires a change in our mindset. Instead of feeling deprived because we are "not allowed" to eat cheap fats, sugars, chemicals, and empty calories, we need to appreciate the beauty of wholesome food and learn how to enjoy the bounty that we are fortunate to have access to in our stores and gardens. We need to learn to *enjoy feeling well*, the result of eating well. And we need to learn to enjoy all of the gloriously colored, antioxidant-rich foods that are available.

12. Remember our ancient ancestors. They ate vastly more leafy greens, wild berries, nuts, and other plants than we do today. They were not exposed to alcohol, refined sugar, empty calories, trans-fats, pesticides, plastics, pollution, cell phones, x-rays, pharmaceutical drugs, nuclear waste, and many of the other causes of oxidative stress. Today, we have stood things on their head: We are exposed to ever-increasing amounts of oxidative stress yet we are eating less and less of the plant foods that will protect us from oxidative stress damage.

THE ULTIMATE SOLUTION: EAT PROPORTIONATE MEALS

Our proportionate meals ensure that at least two-thirds of every meal and snack brings antioxidants into the body. Even when we make poor food choices, if we make our meals proportionate, we will always get antioxidants to help quiet the oxidative stress our "bad" choices generate. When we choose to eat wisely, our grains will be whole and our protein will be nuts, seeds, and beans. Then our whole plate will provide the body with the antioxidants it needs to cope with the oxidative stress generated by the modern world.

VARIETY IS KEY, ANTIOXIDANTS HAVE DIFFERENT PROPERTIES

In a test tube, one antioxidant is equivalent to another. Their ability to reduce (quiet) free radicals in a laboratory setting is often measured and quantified as an ORAC (Oxygen Radical Absorption Capacity) score. Supplements and processed foods are frequently marketed based on their ORAC content. Ads tell us that a serving of noni or açai juice provides 25,000 ORAC units. The implicit message is that we can satisfy our body's antioxidant needs by taking a daily dose of a particular supplement, juice, or food. While these products are rich in antioxidants, our bodies are more complicated than a test tube. We need a variety of antioxidants, more than any given "miracle food" can provide.

Different antioxidants serve different functions in the body and, depending on what is needed at any given moment, getting 25,000 ORAC units of the spectrum of antioxidants in a tropical fruit juice may not provide what we need. Consider the following:

Scurvy is a disease caused by a deficiency of the antioxidant vitamin C. It causes bleeding gums, loss of teeth, and wounds. If a person with scurvy were offered citrus fruit, rich in vitamin C, the scurvy would be cured. On the other hand, if that person were offered avocados with the same ORAC content as the citrus, the scurvy would not be cured: Avocados are high in the antioxidant vitamin E—great for heart health—but they are not famous for their vitamin C content.[6] In a test tube, avocados and citrus will

---

[6] A cup of avocado provides about 12 mg of vitamin C. The same amount of orange provides about 98 mg.

have similar ORAC scores. In the body, they both provide valuable but distinct antioxidants that cannot replace each other.

The poisonous amanita mushroom kills by destroying the liver. In hospitals in Europe, concentrated amounts of milk thistle seed antioxidants are used to prevent the amanita toxins from killing. While a bottle of tropical juice might contain the same amount of ORAC units as the milk thistle antioxidants, the juice would not prevent the mushroom toxins from destroying the liver. In a test tube, these antioxidants are equivalent. In the body, they serve very different functions.

Joint inflammation may be quieted by the curcuminoid antioxidants in turmeric. Lycopene from a tomato might have the same ORAC units of antioxidant power but would not have the same ability to help soothe inflamed joints (lycopene appears to be more beneficial for the prostate). Again, both antioxidants are valuable but serve different functions in the body.

We are just beginning to understand the benefits of the many different antioxidants that a diet rich in plant foods provides. We know that there are some 600 different carotenoids in fruits and vegetables. Beta-carotene, the most famous carotenoid (found in rich amounts in carrots, winter squashes, and sweet potatoes), is important as a precursor to vitamin A. However, the other carotenes (alpha, gamma, delta, epsilon, and zeta) are also important to our health. We know there are at least 4,000 different antioxidants available to us through diet. We do not know exactly what most of these antioxidants do but we do know that they are good for us.

We should be skeptical of claims that an expensive tropical juice, a sweetened chocolate bar, a smoothie, or a supplement can provide anywhere near the benefits of a varied diet delivering a complex mixture of thousands of antioxidant compounds. On occasion, those exotic juices or supplements may serve a purpose: They can be very helpful to a person suffering from influenza or cancer, too sick to eat but in dire need of nutrients. But even then, they need to be chosen wisely and used as a *supplement*, something added to a good diet or used briefly to compensate for an inability to eat well. They will never be able to provide the health benefits of real whole foods and should not be relied on to do so.

As mentioned earlier, a lone antioxidant will on occasion actually increase vulnerability to health issues (such as cancer) where the equivalent antioxidants (in terms of ORAC units) from a varied diet of fruits and vegetables will decrease the risk of cancer.

Finally, we may not be able to absorb and use huge quantities of antioxidants at any given time. Drinking the 25,000 ORAC units in a glass of juice may not provide a greater benefit than eating foods with 20% of that amount: The excess may simply be excreted by the kidneys. Our appetite may well tell us when we have ingested enough of a particular antioxidant.

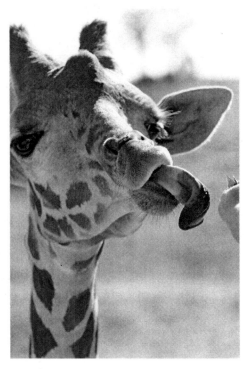

Our goal is to eat as many
different antioxidants as possible

ORAC VALUES OF FRUITS AND VEGETABLES

Fruit, 1 ounce	ORAC	Fruit, 1 ounce	ORAC
Goji (lycii) berry	7,228	Prunes	1,648
Pomegranates	944	Blueberries	685
Blackberries	581	Cranberries	500
Strawberries	440	Raspberries	348
Plums	271	Oranges	241
Grapes, red	211	Cherries	191
Kiwis	174	Grapefruit, pink	141
Grapes, white	131	Cantaloupe	71
Banana	60	Apple	59
Apricot	50	Peach	48
Vegetable, 1 ounce	**ORAC**	**Vegetable, 1 ounce**	**ORAC**
Kale	505	Garlic clove	474
Spinach	360	Yellow squash	328
Brussels sprouts	280	Alfalfa sprouts	265
Steamed spinach	259	Broccoli flowers	254
Beets	240	Avocado	223
Red bell pepper	202	Beans, baked	143
Beans, kidney	131	Onion	128
Corn	114	Eggplant	111
Cauliflower	110	Peas, frozen	107
Potato	85	Sweet potato	84
Cabbage	84	Leaf lettuce	75
Tofu	58	Carrot	57
String beans	57	Tomato	55

Note: One ounce of kale is a very small serving while one ounce of lycii berries may be a reasonable serving. When it comes to vegetables, do not underestimate their antioxidant content and do not underestimate their health benefits.

CHAPTER EIGHT

The Liver's Role

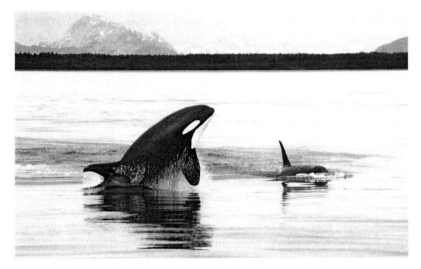

Orca whales have the highest concentration
of PCBs of any creature on earth

According to the Greek physician Hippocrates, the liver is the very core of a healthy body. The liver is vital because it handles so many critical functions: It helps maintain our blood sugar levels. It sorts and processes nutrients from our food, packaging fats and shipping them to parts of the body where they are needed. The liver breaks down excess proteins and prepares them for excretion. The liver is also responsible for detoxifying chemicals we absorb.

While the liver is responsible for detoxification, other organs help excrete toxins. We use our skin (by sweating), our breath (by tiny water droplets), and our kidneys (through urine) for this, but some compounds are also excreted back into the intestines along with bile made in the liver.

Water-soluble compounds are efficiently excreted from the body. However, because fats do not dissolve well in water, they cannot easily travel in water-based urine, sweat, or breath unless attached properly to other water-soluble compounds. Fats are better able to travel out into the intestines along with bile. Yet, if they are not attached properly to the bile, intestinal cells designed to absorb fats quickly pull them back into the body. As a result, when the liver prepares a fat-soluble toxin for excretion (detoxifies), its job is to transform the compound into something that can travel efficiently in water or can be carried out of the body with bile and not be reabsorbed.

Most troublesome toxins are fat-soluble, and enter the body in the fats in our food. Our liver uses enzymes to attach toxins to water-soluble compounds, and we are able to excrete many toxins that way. However, the liver is less successful when handling man-made, fat-soluble toxins that are "persistent" and "accumulate up the food chain." We do not have detoxification systems for these recently developed toxins and our livers (and those of other animals) are unable to efficiently transform these chemicals into an excretable form. These toxins accumulate in our bodies because we cannot efficiently excrete them.

As these toxic chemicals are processed in the liver, or are periodically released from our fat cells and recirculated in our bodies, they cause damage in a variety of ways that we will discuss later in this chapter. First, however, we are going to discuss some of the persistent toxins that currently *all of us* carry in our bodies, old and young alike.

Because we cannot efficiently excrete these toxins, each of us carries a toxin load (an accumulated quantity) of a variety of chemicals. The Toxic-Free Legacy Coalition of the State of Washington sampled toxin loads in ten volunteers, including a breast cancer surgeon, a fundraiser for breast cancer research, a public health nurse, two Washington state senators, and an environmental activist. All tested positive for 29 persistent toxins and heavy metals. The environmental activist—who ate only organically grown food—had no pesticides in her blood but still carried many, many other toxins.

Neither animals nor humans are able to efficiently rid their bodies of persistent toxins, and these toxins accumulate up the food chain. Plants absorb small amounts of environmental toxins. When a small animal eats plants, any toxins in them are added to the toxins the animal has already consumed. When a larger animal consumes the smaller animal, the larger animal absorbs all of the toxins stored in the smaller animal. For example, chickens eat feed laced with persistent chemicals. We eat the first chicken and get (and retain) all its toxins; we eat a second chicken and get (and retain) all its toxins. We cannot excrete the toxins, hence they "accumulate."

SOME WELL-KNOWN PERSISTENT TOXINS
DDT

DDT is a fat-soluble chemical that accumulates up the food chain. Once inside our body, the liver converts some of the DDT to DDD and DDE, two yet more toxic compounds. We are able to excrete some of this DDD and DDE. The liver does not efficiently convert the remaining DDT. In fact, it has a half-life (the length of time taken to expel one-half of the remaining DDT) of a lifetime. In other words, once we absorb DDT, much of it will remain with us for the rest of our lives. The only time such a fat-soluble persistent toxin is easily released from the body is when a woman breastfeeds. (DDT and other toxins travel on the fat in breast milk into the infant's body, reducing the mother's toxic load.)

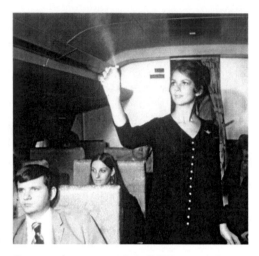

Stewardess spraying DDT on a plane.

While DDT use is on the decline, it persists in the food chain because of its long half-life. In addition, while we are exposed to less DDT today than in years past, our use of other persistent toxins is increasing faster than DDT is declining.

PCBs

PCBs (polychlorinated biphenyls) consist of groups of chlorinated chemicals. PCBs were used to cool electrical transformers to avert explosions. Haphazard dumping of old transformers led to pervasive environmental contamination over a period of many years. PCBs now are concentrated in wildlife and are accumulating up the food chain. Orca whales have the highest concentration of any creature on earth. One of those PCBs has a half-life of 28 years. So if our fish dinner contains that particular PCB, 28 years later we will have cleared *half* of that specific PCB from our body.

FLAME RETARDANTS

Environmental contamination from flame retardants is rising rapidly. Orcas and dolphins contain concentrated amounts because their diet consists of fish, and most fish now are contaminated with flame retardants. Fish are contaminated because flame retardant–treated carpets, car upholstery, furniture, clothes, and other articles are disposed of in landfills that leach the chemicals into the water. We also spray forest fires with flame retardants. Rainfall and runoff deliver these chemicals through the water supply to the fish.

Fish historically have been a very healthy food providing high amounts of omega-3 fats and, if fatty, also vitamin D. (People living in Northern latitudes once survived periods of little or no sunlight by eating large amounts of fish.) However, it is no longer recommended that we eat seafood daily. As seafood becomes more contaminated with persistent toxins and heavy metals, we must balance its inherent benefits against its acquired detriments such as flame retardants and mercury. Farmed fish often are so high in flame retardants that some recommend that we not eat farmed Atlantic salmon more than once a month.

PHTHALATES

Phthalates are highly reactive chemicals found in certain plastics. Bisphenol-A (BPA), the chemical presently raising the most concern, is often found in baby bottles, water bottles, intravenous ("IV") drip bags, sealants for children's teeth, and the lining in canned foods. BPA leaches out of those products and into our bodies where it persists and accumulates. We may also be absorbing significant amounts of this chemical from heat-treated credit card receipts. A recent study found that many heat-set cash register receipts are covered with significant amounts of BPA. In fact, plastic water bottles that leach nanograms of BPA are considered a problem. In contrast, cash register receipts may expose us to milligrams of BPA. One milligram is equal to a million nanograms.

PERFLUORINATED CHEMICALS

Another growing problem involves contamination from "perfluorinated chemicals." These chemicals are found in teflon, non-stick cookware, stain-resistant textiles, and food packaging. Packaging is treated with these chemicals to prevent greasy foods from soaking through the packaging. Unfortunately, the perfluorinated chemicals in the packaging are rapidly absorbed by the fats in the food and travel with the food into our bodies.

Popcorn bags, pizza boxes, candy wrappers, and the little bags and boxes that hold french fries and burgers are examples of packaging that pose this problem. We even get a smidgen of perfluorinated chemicals from certain brands of non-stick dental floss.

HEAVY METALS

Animals and humans also have problems excreting heavy metals such as mercury, cadmium, arsenic, and lead. Today, pregnant women and children are told to not eat too much tuna and other large fish because they contain significant amounts of mercury. Mercury poses a problem for all humans and mercury is pervasive. It was found in high levels in both sushi tuna at fancy New York restaurants and regular canned tuna. We are also exposed to mercury as a contaminant found in many high-fructose corn syrups.

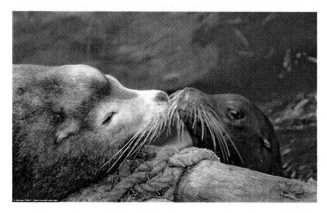

Sea lions dying from bladder cancer have
unusually high PCB loads

How toxins damage

Each of the persistent toxins damages the body, and especially the liver, in a variety of ways. For instance, the FDA recently concluded that BPA can damage the heart. PCBs suppress the immune system. Sea lions are increasingly dying of aggressive bladder cancers. Cancerous sea lions have higher concentrations of PCBs than healthy sea lions. Experts believe that these PCBs suppress the sea lions' immune system and make them more vulnerable to cancer-causing viruses. Many of these persistent toxins disrupt our hormone balances. One troubling way they harm us is by mimicking the action of human estrogen, a xenoestrogenic effect, described next.

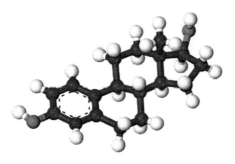

Estradiol

Human estrogen

Estrogen is a female reproductive hormone, but all humans (men, women, and children) have cells that can bind and respond to estrogen. Adult women make three different types of estrogen. During a woman's reproductive years, estradiol, a strong estrogen, is the most prevalent form of estrogen. During pregnancy, women produce estriol, a weaker estrogen. Post-menopausal women circulate a yet weaker form of estrogen, estrone.

Estrogen has many actions in a woman's body but its primary function is to trigger growth of certain tissues. During periods of a month when a woman produces more estradiol, the hormone causes breast and uterine tissue to proliferate. The tissue is used to form milk ducts needed to nurse a baby and to form the placenta for a growing fetus. This action is referred to as an *estrogenic effect*.

Many types of cells (breast, uterine, prostate, bone, and brain, to name a few) have receptors that can bind estrogen. These receptors are found on cells in women, men, and children. Men make small amounts of estrogen as their bodies process testosterone. While men and children have estrogen receptors, they are not designed to have much estrogen circulating that might bind to those cell receptors. However, there are many man-made, estrogen-like compounds that are present in our environment today that can bind to those receptors. These are called xenoestrogens.

WHAT ARE XENOESTROGENS?

Many persistent toxins are "xenoestrogens." Xeno comes from a Greek word that means foreign. Xenoestrogens are man-made chemicals that have an estrogenic effect. Xenoestrogens bind to estrogen receptors on cells and usually trigger a strong estrogenic effect. This is especially problematic for males and young girls. Men, boys, and young girls (or the equivalent in other species) are not supposed to have many estrogenic compounds in their bodies, and any estrogen they do have should be very weak.

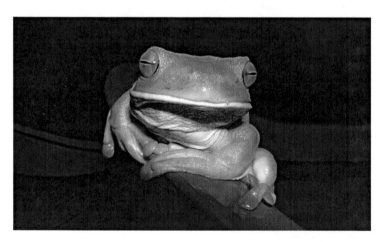

Frogs are very sensitive to toxins

Today, all of us have xenoestrogens circulating in our bodies and we are starting to see their xenoestrogenic effect manifest as reproductive chaos: Male salmon are turning female as they age.

Male halibut are laying eggs. Male frogs are born with multiple testes and also have multiple ovaries. Norwegian scientists found hermaphroditic polar bears. In male humans, we are seeing increases in testicular cancer, sperm abnormalities, lowered sperm counts, and male breast cancer. Young girls are reaching puberty at earlier ages. While still very rare, there are girls who have entered puberty at age one. More common is the early onset of some aspects of puberty, where girls develop breasts and pubic hair as early as age four but do not begin menstruating until age eight, nine, or ten.

The rise in breast cancer, ovarian cancer, premenstrual problems, fertility issues, and the difficult menopausal transition that adult women increasingly experience are likely due in large part to xenoestrogens. Xenoestrogens are also problematic in anyone with an estrogen-sensitive cancer.[1]

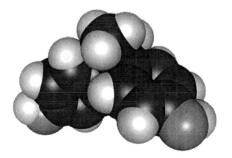

Bisphenol-A is xenoestrogenic

BPA (the chemical used in plastic bottles and on cash register receipts) is a xenoestrogen. DDE (a breakdown product of DDT), PCBs, BHA (butylated hydroxyanisole, a food preservative), and dieldrin (a now-banned insecticide) are also xenoestrogens.

---

[1] Of course, the chemical industry vigorously denies any and all such effects, claiming a lack of scientific evidence. They also claim that many xenoestrogens only have a weak estrogenic effect. This debate will continue into the future. At best—and highly unlikely given the results we see in the world around us—persistent chemicals might prove harmless. No one claims that they hold any benefit whatsoever in the body.

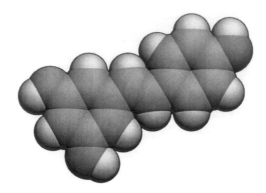

Resveratrol in red wine is a phytoestrogen

COMBATING XENOESTROGENS WITH PHYTOESTROGENS

We all carry a load of xenoestrogens in our bodies because they are environmental toxins we cannot completely avoid and cannot efficiently detoxify and excrete. At present, our main defense against this estrogenic load comes from another group of estrogen-like compounds: Phytoestrogens.

Phytoestrogens are estrogenic compounds made by plants. They too bind to estrogen receptors on cells, but typically trigger a very weak estrogenic effect. We have evolved eating foods rich in phytoestrogens and are well-adapted to their effects. Examples of phytoestrogens include resveratrol found in red wine, quercetin found in onions and watermelon, lignans found in flax seed, and isoflavones such as genistein and daidzein found in soy and other beans.[2]

HOW PHYTOESTROGENS BENEFIT US

Estrogens are constantly binding to cell receptors, triggering an estrogenic effect. They bind, are released, and then bind to the receptor again. In a body filled with both estrogens and xenoestrogens, the chemicals compete for these binding sites. It

---

[2] The phytoestrogens in beans, for example soybeans, are among the strongest of phytoestrogens. In isolated form, they may be equivalent to estradiol in strength. However, combined with other compounds in beans, their estrogenic effect appears to be quite different—and weaker—than that of estradiol and xenoestrogens.

is a bit like a game of musical chairs. If one or the other type is present in greater amounts, that type will most often succeed in binding to the cell and having an effect on the body.

Phytoestrogens may be one of our best defenses against xenoestrogens. They too bind to estrogen receptors and compete in this game of musical chairs. When they "win," we experience less of an estrogenic effect. Consider a young child who has accumulated xenoestrogens from the time he or she was in the uterus: Phytoestrogens in that child's diet will compete with xenoestrogens for estrogen receptors on his or her cells. If phytoestrogens are plentiful, they will win the race for binding sites more often than not. When they do, only a very weak signal is sent to the cell to multiply or grow. On the other hand, if few phytoestrogens are in the child's diet, the xenoestrogens will "win" every time, sending a strong estrogenic message to the cells in the child's body. Thus phytoestrogens may lessen the effect of xenoestrogens.

Today all—men, women, and children—have accumulated xenoestrogens. We gain a degree of protection from them by eating large amounts of plant foods and filling our bodies with phytoestrogens.[3]

PERSISTENT TOXINS DISRUPT OTHER HORMONES

Most research on persistent toxins has focused on their estrogenic effect. Increasingly, however, studies show that these chemicals also affect other hormone systems. Persistent chemicals bind to a variety of receptor sites throughout our bodies—sometimes enhancing, sometimes blocking, the normal function of our hormones. Others interfere with the breakdown of hormones or the rate of their synthesis. Important hormone systems that are affected include thyroid hormone (which affects metabolism), the

---

[3] Our preagricultural ancestors ate a diet rich in phytoestrogens. They ate more foods containing phytoestrogens and had more of those compounds in their bodies than people have today. They were not exposed to xenoestrogens. Females often were in a pregnant, low-estrogenic state, and our ancestors were exposed to vastly less estrogenic messaging than the cleanest living person today.

glucocorticoid system (disruption of this system is associated with autoimmune disease, non–insulin dependent diabetes, and obesity), testosterone (a male reproductive hormone), and progesterone (a female reproductive hormone).

Persistent toxins are environmental toxins, meaning that they are found all across the globe, and we cannot escape them. They concentrate up the food chain so the larger the animal, the greater its toxin load. We are high on the food chain and accumulate large amounts of these toxins. We cannot efficiently rid our bodies of them once they are in us. Instead, along with increasing our intake of phytoestrogens, we need to work on avoiding or reducing the amount of persistent toxins in our diet.

How food choices help us avoid persistent toxins

Animal products are one of our main sources of persistent toxins. Today, 100% of beef still tests positive for DDT. Cheese, bologna, ice cream, hot dogs, and other animal products (foods we often feed our children) contain DDT (94% tested positive). Because DDT is an environmental toxin, it will be found in both factory-farmed and grass-fed animal products.[4] And, as DDT dwindles away, other persistent toxins are rapidly taking its place and contaminating our foods.

Many weight-loss diets recommend eating a large amount of protein based on a conjecture that our ancient ancestors ate a great deal of animal protein. The debate continues about the amount of animal protein actually in their diet,[5] but what is indisputable is that their animal products did not carry man-made toxic chemicals. Today, because our world is polluted, we cannot limit our exposure to toxins and simultaneously continue to eat large quantities of meat, dairy, poultry, and seafood products.

We should be particularly concerned about what we feed our children. Grandparents born in the early part of the 20th century

---

[4] Of course, organic or 100% grass-fed animals will contain vastly fewer toxins than factory-farmed animals but they nonetheless provide environmental toxins.

[5] While hunter/gatherers certainly ate more animals than grains, it is much less clear that they ate more animals than non-grain plants.

were exposed to minimal amounts of toxins as children. Their children, born mid-century, were first exposed to xenoestrogens and other persistent toxins as adults. Children today, however, are exposed to them from the moment of conception. Because the use of toxic compounds continues to increase, our children's exposure over a lifetime will be yet greater than ever before. If we want to give them the foundation for healthy, long lives, and if they are to be able to provide us with healthy grandchildren, we need to limit their intake of persistent toxins. We need to teach them to eat well both by serving healthy meals but also by setting a good example with our own diet. If not, we run the risk of compromising their health, their reproductive abilities including their ability to produce and breastfeed their own children.

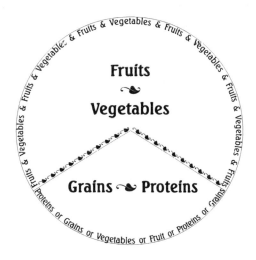

The proportionate meal helps us cope with environmental toxins. First, we limit the proportion of animal protein in our meals. Second, every meal and snack provides a significant amount of fruits and vegetables, ensuring that our diet is rich in phytoestrogens and other plant nutrients that help our bodies cope with these chemicals. As we become aware of the problems of persistent toxins, we can increasingly serve (and eat) meals that are "lower on the food chain." When we eat nuts and beans instead of animal protein, we significantly reduce our intake of toxins while increasing our intake of phytoestrogens.

REDUCE TOXIN EXPOSURE

We also should work on avoiding chemicals in and around our home. For instance, we can avoid foods stored in treated packaging and can save leftovers in glass rather than plastic containers. Each and every chemical that we replace with a less toxic chemical, or that we eliminate, lessens the magnitude of our toxic load. Certainly, we should refuse to buy foods with added chemicals and instead only eat real, whole foods. We also need to evaluate our exposure to chemicals such as insecticides and fungicides.

PESTICIDES: INSECTICIDES, HERBICIDES, AND FUNGICIDES

Many of the chemicals applied to food crops are persistent and/or xenoestrogenic. Although our government assures us that the remaining pesticide residues are safe, studies are beginning to contradict those assurances: One study found that children eating berries sprayed with organophosphate pesticides had a much higher incidence of attention-deficit/hyperactivity disorder (ADHD). We can avoid pesticide residues by eating only organically-grown food but many of us cannot afford the extra cost of organic foods. We can, however, try to avoid the produce most likely to carry the heaviest pesticide residue. If we avoid them we can cut our pesticide intake in half, a significant amount. We can also eat more of the produce least likely to have pesticide residues.

Consumer groups have created lists identifying the most and least contaminated produce was compiled. These lists help us avoid chemicals on our foods but they are not perfect:

First, they report on amounts of pesticide residue on the food, not the relative toxicity of each pesticide. The toxicity of pesticides varies; a small residue of a far more toxic pesticide may be worse for us than a larger amount of a less toxic chemical. These lists do not consider this fact.

Second, onions always are included in the "clean" lists and are seldom sprayed (althouth one study found that 24% of all fungicides were used on onions). However, conventional onions along with potatoes, garlic, and other bulbs, are treated after harvest with anti-sprouting agents. These agents are not regulated as carefully as pesticides. Some scientists urge great caution with anti-sprouting agents because those chemicals are tampering with turning cell growth on-and-off, the hallmark of cancer.

Dirty Dozen	Clean Dozen
Celery	Asparagus
Peaches	Avocado
Strawberries	Cabbage
Apples	Cantaloupe (U.S.)
Blueberries	Eggplant
Nectarines	Kiwi (tropical)
Peppers	Mango
Spinach	Onions
Kale/Collards	Pineapple
Cherries	Sweet Corn (frozen)
Potatoes	Sweet Peas (frozen)
Grapes (imported)	Watermelon

One of the best ways to determine which foods to avoid in conventional form is to visit the website http://www.whatsonmyfood. org/food.jsp?food=BB and look at the actual chemicals found on the food you are considering buying. Along with the frequency of residue, this site lists the chemicals found and the safety concerns they may pose.

We should be especially careful about exposing our children to chemicals. The government does attempt to set pesticide residues at a safe level but children will often eat large amounts of cherries, berries, grapes, raisins, peaches, and other foods they are fond of. They may end up ingesting more residue than the government took into account. Moreover, children's bodies are still developing and they are more sensitive to the effect of these chemicals than adults are.

PRODUCE SOAPS

Another recommended way to avoid pesticides is to peel or wash produce with soaps that are able to remove non–water-soluble chemicals. This does not always work.

During the early stages of industrialized agriculture, chemicals were sprayed on growing plants to kill insects. Today, many pesticides are systemic. They are sprayed on the soil and the plant absorbs them. These chemicals are not intended to kill the insects outright; instead, they are intended to thwart insect reproduction. These chemicals are called endocrine disruptors, another expression for chemicals that designed to cause reproductive chaos the way xenoestrogens do. It is a good idea to wash or peel conventional produce, just in case they carry a topical residue, but we cannot assume that the wash will solve our problems—in many cases it will not.

CONVENTIONAL PRODUCE IS STILL GOOD FOR US

The purpose of this discussion is not meant to cast us into despair or to frighten the wits out of us. The purpose is instead to emphasize the importance of avoiding as many chemicals as we can. It highlights the benefits of organically-grown foods; if we can afford them, they are worth the extra money. But many of us cannot. In that case, we need to remember that fruits and vegetables are *extremely* good for us, even with their chemical residues.

This is analogous to human breast milk. The human toxin load is so high that all breast milk is filled with persistent toxins. Nonetheless, it without question remains the best food for an infant. The good in the milk vastly outweighs the problems those chemicals may pose. Similarly, fruits and vegetables contain many, many compounds that protect our health and are vital to us. Thus, even conventionally grown produce provides benefits that absolutely and vastly outweigh any chemical residue in or on them.

SIMPLE STEPS WE SHOULD TAKE TO AVOID TOXINS

We cannot avoid all environmental toxins but we can learn more about them, the problems they pose, and how better to avoid them.[6] We can also take simple steps to protect our children and ourselves:

---

[6] A good place to begin learning about them is the website at http://www. watoxics.org/chemicals-of-concern/perfluorinated-compounds-pfcs

We can encourage our children to eat lower on the food chain. Help them, for example, choose nuts over string cheese, and fruit over ice cream.

We can reduce the amount of animal products in our diet and increase the amount of fruits and vegetables.

We can grow some of our own food, whether in a big garden or in a few pots.

We can shop locally from farmers who do not use chemicals.

Having done what we can in that respect, we should make sure that we support our livers as they process the toxins we cannot avoid.

WAYS TO SUPPORT AND STRENGTHEN THE LIVER

Our livers are continuously exposed to damaging chemicals as they enter and circulate in our bodies. In addition to reducing our exposure to them, we should do as much as we can to protect our livers from their damage:

TAKE HOT BATHS, SAUNAS, SWEAT

Hot baths, a soak in a hot tub, a sauna, or working up a sweat helps move toxins out of the body. These pleasurable activities, unfortunately, will not move persistent toxins out of our body but these "treatments" will speed up the removal of water-soluble toxins and waste. In turn, this frees the liver to more quickly process the more difficult toxins and store them away where they do less damage.

EAT MORE BERRIES

Eat lots of berries, the wilder and darker the better. Berries are rich in powerful antioxidants that are particularly good at preventing chemicals from damaging the body.

EAT MORE GREEN VEGETABLES

Leafy greens and cruciferous vegetables (e.g., broccoli, Brussels sprouts, cauliflower,) contain compounds that the liver uses in its detoxification system. They also contain compounds that protect the liver from damage as it processes toxins.

EAT MORE ONIONS AND GARLIC

Eat onions and garlic frequently. Their sulfurous compounds help the liver detoxify chemicals and prevent toxin damage.

EAT MUSHROOMS, FERMENTED FOODS, AND SEAWEED

Include mushrooms, fermented plant foods (e.g, miso, sauerkraut, kimchee), and seaweed in your diet. These foods are especially good at growing interesting strains of beneficial microbes. Our good microbes bind toxins in our food and prevent us from absorbing them. The benefit of well-balanced intestinal flora should not be underestimated. This is also a reason to be careful with treatments that purport to "cleanse" the colon using methods that wash out or starve our beneficial flora.

USE CITRUS PEEL

Use organic citrus peel in your food and beverages. Citrus peel contains many compounds that reduce toxin damage. It may be that we add citrus slivers to cocktails because we know intuitively that it will offset or reduce the damage alcohol can cause.

FORAGE

Learn to eat wild greens such as nettles, dandelion, and purslane. Many wild greens are bitter, and their bitter taste stimulates liver function. Wild greens also contain unusual compounds that help the liver detoxify.

Consider milk thistle: While milk thistle is often listed as a noxious weed, it has rather remarkable health benefits. In Europe, antioxidants (silymarin) found in milk thistle seeds are concentrated and used in emergency rooms to prevent the poisonous amanita mushroom from destroying the liver. A number of ongoing clinical studies are testing silymarin's ability to help those suffering from liver cancer, hepatitis, and skin cancers.

Milk thistle seeds actually contain only tiny amounts of silymarin. Nonetheless, Russian studies indicate that ground milk thistle seed used in baking—or simmered as a tea—helps protect the liver.

The message is not to run out and buy milk thistle supplements. Instead, the message is that we should eat more of the "weeds" that our foraging ancestors ate. Many gardeners have a long-standing battle with the weed purslane—a green vegetable with the highest amount of omega-3 fats of any land plant. We should pick and eat it instead of trying to kill it. We should pick wild berries which are much higher in omega-3 fats than their cultivated cousins. We should eat some of our bitter dandelion leaves instead of spraying them with herbicides. Dandelion leaf has a long-standing folk reputation as a liver protectant. Try some of the more exotic, wild mushrooms offered at the store as a change from the little button mushrooms. These are but a few examples of wild foods that we could bring back into our diet, at least occasionally.

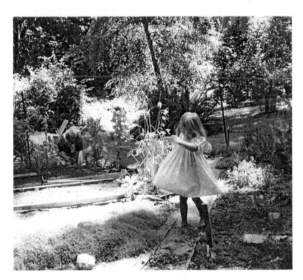

Dancing and gardening help both liver and spirit

Move more

Move. Do not make a grim resolution to join a gym and endure exercise to lose weight but instead move more to stimulate metabolic activity. Start to see physical activity from the viewpoint of how it will help the liver. This makes walking, dancing, gardening, or any movement more approachable. When we move, we generate glutathione, a very important compound for the body and for liver health (see chapter 18). And, remember, if pain, excess weight, or a busy schedule prevent you from exercising, compensate with more antioxidants and far fewer empty calories.

Chapter summary

We can help our bodies cope with environmental chemicals. If we eat lower on the food chain, eat unsprayed foods when possible, and avoid chemicals in our food and home, we reduce our exposure to toxins. If we eat proportionately and fill the protein/ grain portion of our plate with more nuts, seeds, beans, and whole grains, we increase our intake of phytoestrogens. If we take hot baths or saunas, eat more berries, eat more green vegetables, onions, garlic, mushrooms, fermented foods, and seaweeds, use citrus peel, eat some wilder foods, and move more, we will be better able to handle the toxins we cannot avoid.

CHAPTER NINE
Insulin Resistance

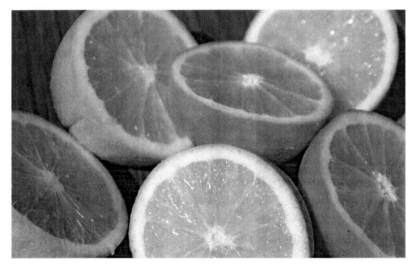

Juice increases the risk of diabetes.

One of the liver's many functions is to help maintain normal glucose (or blood sugar) levels. This is a vital function because the brain requires a steady supply of the right amount of glucose. Excessive amounts of glucose can cause confusion and coma. Too little can cause seizures, brain damage, and death. Even moderate blood sugar imbalances have a negative effect on the brain.

THE INSULIN/GLUCAGON "SEESAW"

When we eat, we absorb sugar from our intestines into our bloodstream and our blood sugar levels rise. Whenever our blood sugar level rises above the normal range (hyperglycemia), the pancreas secretes the hormone insulin. Insulin tells the liver and muscles to remove the extra sugar from the blood and store it away as glycogen. This causes the blood sugar level to move back into the normal range again. As it does, insulin release slows.

We use blood sugar as a source of quick energy. We use it to move around, breathe, and think. As we burn energy, our blood sugar levels begin to drop below the normal range (hypoglycemia). When blood sugar levels drop, the pancreas secretes a different hormone, glucagon. Glucagon signals the liver to convert stored glycogen back to glucose and release it into the bloodstream.[1] As blood sugar levels return to the normal range, the pancreas slows glucagon release.

Thus, insulin and glucagon take turns rising and falling to ensure our blood sugar levels stay within a safe range, neither too high nor too low, so we have a steady supply of blood sugar for our physical and mental activity. This seesaw system of insulin and glucagon works well if we eat appropriately.

The average Western diet, however, does not allow this interplay

---

[1] When needed, glucagon also tells the liver to make glucose from other types of stored energy, such as fats.

of insulin and glucagon to function as it should. Too often, we eat "high-glycemic" foods (cookies, for example) that quickly raise, or spike, our blood sugar to high levels. In response, larger amounts of insulin are released to quickly bring our blood sugar levels back to the safe range where we thrive. However, that extra insulin (released in response to the spike in blood sugar) takes longer to leave the bloodstream. This residual insulin prevents an effective release of glucagon from the pancreas when our blood sugar drops. The liver does not receive the signal to break down stored glycogen and release it as we use up our blood sugar. Without the right ratio of insulin to glucagon, the liver does not effectively maintain our blood sugar levels and cannot act to prevent hypoglycemia as we use up the sugar in the blood.

The brain needs a steady supply of blood sugar to function. It responds to hypoglycemia by triggering food cravings, usually for foods that spike blood sugar levels. So we eat another high-glycemic meal or snack. Once again, our blood sugar spikes and insulin levels spike to match. We enter into a cycle where insulin and glucagon no longer play seesaw with each other. Instead, we are stuck in a dance of unstable blood sugar levels, residual insulin, food cravings, and grazing.

With time, due to sugar spikes, overeating, and eating too often, our muscles and liver cells become saturated with glycogen. They do not have "room" to store more. Eventually, liver and muscle cells quit responding to insulin and do not absorb glucose from the blood. They become "insulin-resistant." We still must maintain normal blood sugar levels. When the liver and muscles become resistant, insulin instead triggers fat cells to absorb the excess glucose and store it as fat.

Because the liver is not breaking down glycogen effectively, blood sugar levels are often out of the normal range. It becomes difficult to go without food for any length of time or even to sleep through the night. Bedtime snacks become irresistible. Because more glucose is sent to fat storage, weight gain occurs at a faster rate.

Over time, the fat cells also fatigue. They too become insulin-resistant in response to the constant barrage of messages from insulin. It takes higher and higher levels of insulin to get the fat cells to absorb excess blood sugar. In order to maintain appropriate blood sugar levels, the individual must secrete ever larger amounts of insulin. This creates a vicious cycle if the individual does not make lifestyle changes.

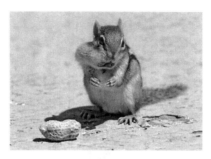

We do not nibble between
meals and snacks.

Eating too frequently also stresses the pancreas. In between meals, the pancreas prepares and stores a form of insulin that is secreted as a "first response" to rising blood sugar levels after a meal. Additional insulin is secreted in a second phase. Constant snacking inhibits storage of "first response" insulin, leading to an exaggerated second phase secretion of insulin. This burdens the pancreas.

Eventually, blood sugar control begins to falter. In the pre-diabetic state, it takes longer and longer for blood sugar levels to return to normal after a meal. The person spends more time in a hyperglycemic state. Eventually, the body cannot produce enough insulin to return blood sugar levels to normal and the person becomes a type 2 (non–insulin dependent) diabetic. Although the person's pancreas still secretes insulin, the cells require ever higher levels of insulin before they respond. The pancreas can no longer produce enough insulin to achieve normal blood sugar levels. The individual now needs prescription oral diabetes drugs to maintain normal blood sugar levels.[2]

---

[2] Type 2 diabetes is quite common and current estimates are that one out of every three adults will be diabetic by the year 2050.

If this individual continues to eat poorly, the pancreas will continue to overproduce insulin until at some point the pancreatic cells burn out and no longer make adequate amounts of insulin. At that point, the individual will have to use insulin injections to maintain normal blood sugar levels.

REPAIRING THE INSULIN/GLUCAGON RESPONSE

On this plan, we work to overcome insulin resistance and help our liver maintain healthy blood sugar levels in two distinct ways:

First, we have times when we eat (meals and snacks) as well as periods of time where we eat nothing that triggers an insulin response. While we may have coffee with a whitener (such as nut or soy milk) with our breakfast, when we leave the breakfast table, we leave that whitened coffee behind. In between meals and snacks we do not drink anything except black coffee, plain tea, herbal tea, or water. We do not nibble little bits of food—no grapes, nuts, mints, or other bites of food. We do not even chew sugarless gum. We do not eat again until the next meal or snack.

We have our five meals a day but nothing in between them. And, after dinner, we quit eating two to three hours before bed. This creates a long overnight fast. These breaks will help end the insulin dominance and restore the insulin glucagon seesaw so the liver is able to respond to glucagon again.

At first, many of us have a hard time not grazing. We are used to maintaining our energy levels (actually our blood sugar levels) by constantly snacking. We can become fatigued, jittery, or out-of-sorts if we do not plan our meals and snacks carefully. Our bodies quickly metabolize fruits and vegetables and about an hour after eating them, the energy they contain has been absorbed, used, or stored in the body. At that point, we have to rely on our liver to maintain our blood sugar levels for the next hour or two until snack time. Often, the liver is not prepared for this job. Therefore, we must make sure that we eat enough food and, more importantly, more complex foods in the form of protein and fats. Fats are metabolized slowly; it may take two to three hours to absorb and store their components. Fats help "carry" us from meal to snack, and from snack to meal.

This is also why snacks are important: Often we get busy during the day and do not want to stop and have a snack. However, if we do not, we may begin to develop blood sugar yo-yos that, in turn, will trigger food cravings and make it very hard to eat properly.

> ### THE DETOX REACTION
>
> Sometimes the sense of fatigue, headaches, and malaise—comonly called a detox reaction—is simply the body adapting to normal blood sugar levels. Pre-diabetic and diabetic individuals often report that normal blood sugar levels (after a period of higher levels) cause uncomfortable sensations that take a while to dissipate. Take heart, this too will pass.

The second way we can work on overcoming insulin resistance is by increasing the amount of green vegetables in our diet. Chloroplasts contain chlorophyll which also can help us overcome insulin resistance because green vegetables make our cells more responsive to insulin. If our cells are more sensitive to insulin, we need less insulin to achieve normal blood sugar levels.[3] The less circulating insulin we have, the quicker our insulin levels can return to normal after the excess glucose is removed from the blood. As our insulin levels normalize, glucagon can come into play again. Our green vegetables are important allies in maintaining normal blood sugar levels because they make cells more sensitive, more responsive, to insulin.

It is fine to eat fruits—they contain fiber and many nutrients—but fruits do not help us overcome insulin resistance. In reasonable amounts, fruits are neutral in this regard. Excess fructose from any other source, however, will increase insulin resistance. That is why women who drank a glass of orange juice a day—instead of eating

---

[3] Increased sensitivity is one reason that individuals taking oral diabetes medications or using insulin often need to reduce their doses of these medications when they follow the TQI diet. Increased insulin sensitivity is helpful even in cases where the pancreas does not produce adequate amounts of insulin.

whole fruit—ended up with an 18 percent higher incidence of diabetes. It is also why eating excess fructose may double the rate of systolic hypertension (high blood pressure where the top number rises, a form of high blood pressure more common in the elderly).

We tend to get too much fructose when we drink juices. And, because we usually eliminate the fiber from our juice, the juice raises our blood sugar levels much more quickly than does the same amount of fruit. Other forms of fructose, including large amounts of dried fruit, agave nectar, and high-fructose corn syrup, increase insulin resistance, and need to be avoided.

MAINTAINING HEALTHY BLOOD SUGAR LEVELS

Once the seesaw game between insulin and glucagon is back in play, your liver will do a fine job of maintaining your blood sugar levels between meals. At that point, you may find that you can omit snacks without experiencing food cravings, headaches, or moodiness. You may then choose to eliminate snacks.

You must continue to eat a healthy diet, free of the sugars and refined foods that interfere with proper metabolic hormone function. Resist grazing and night eating, and eat several servings of chlorophyll-containing vegetables every day. And remember, healing the body and restoring full liver function may take time. Some commentators suggest that anyone who is five or more pounds overweight is insulin-resistant to some degree. If you have a degree of insulin resistance and quit eating snacks, you put yourself at higher risk for sudden food cravings that can be hard to resist, so continuing to eat small snacks is often a wise decision.

If you are a non–insulin dependent diabetic, you may find that your blood sugar levels vary too much over night if you do not have a bedtime snack. You should first and foremost focus on maintaining safe glucose levels. You may need a bedtime snack. Later, as your health improves, you can experiment to see if you can eliminate the bedtime snack from your diet. If you are an insulin-dependent diabetic, you likely will always need to eat at bedtime.

GLYCEMIC LOAD AND INSULIN RESPONSE

Most plans targeting insulin resistance and blood sugar control focus on the glycemic index of foods. While the glycemic index is of value, it is not as valuable as many assume.

The glycemic index was created to rank foods according to how quickly they increase blood glucose levels. However, in quieting inflammation *how* foods may increase the release of insulin is of equal—or greater—importance. For instance, white bread is higher on the glycemic index than whole grain bread but both trigger a similar amount of insulin release. Most fruits are much lower on the glycemic index than pasta and bread (even white bread) but fruits trigger more insulin. Carbohydrates are high on the glycemic index but other foods, lower on that index, also increase insulin secretion. Protein-rich foods or protein combined with carbohydrates can stimulate insulin production without increasing (and sometimes decreasing) blood sugar levels, nonetheless triggering an inflammatory effect.

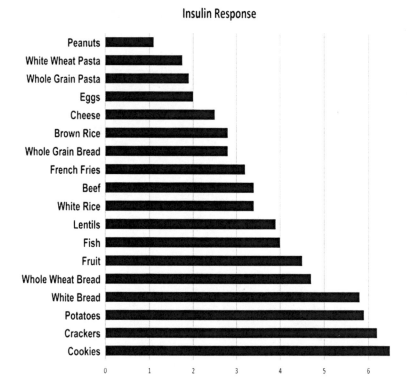

Insulin Response

It turns out that the relationship between glycemic index and the insulin response is not linear. We need more than a table of the glycemic index of foods if we are to make good food choices that moderate our insulin response. We also need to consider how nutritious the food is. For instance, a low carb Atkins bar produces an insulin response almost equal to white bread. Neither one is an antioxidant-rich whole food and neither feeds the beneficial intestinal flora. Wild fish evokes more insulin than beef does but is more nutritious because it provides omega-3 fats. Beef and cheese cause a lower insulin response than lentils but are less nutritious because they contain saturated fats and toxins but do not contain antioxidants or fiber.

On the TQI Diet, we eat a variety of high-glycemic vegetables (yams, sweet potatoes, carrots, etc.) because they are rich in antioxidants, other plant nutrients, and fiber. We are mindful of the glycemic index and combine those vegetables with other foods to reduce their tendency to spike our blood sugar. We do not, however, limit or eliminate healthy foods based solely on measurements of glycemic index, glycemic load, and insulin response. Instead, our goal is to choose foods that provide the greatest anti-inflammatory benefit (e.g., whole fruits and vegetables, legumes, seeds, nuts, and fish).

EXCESS INSULIN IS INFLAMMATORY

Excess sugar in the diet increases the amount of insulin released. Excess insulin in our blood prevents another hormone, glucagon, from functioning as it should (see discussion above). But insulin does more than simply regulate the uptake of glucose by cells; it also causes cells to store nutrients not needed for immediate use.

As insulin resistance takes hold in the body, the cells decrease their uptake of magnesium. The magnesium we should have stored for future use is instead lost in the urine. Intracellular magnesium relaxes all types of muscles, and our blood vessels are surrounded by a layer of muscle tissue. As we eat sugar, release insulin, and lose magnesium in the urine, the muscles around our blood vessels constrict. As they constrict, our blood pressure rises.

Excess insulin also causes the body to retain sodium. In turn, we retain fluid which also causes blood pressure to rise.

Most of us do not eat diets sufficiently rich in magnesium to begin with. We aggravate this problem by eating a diet rich in sugars, causing the loss of the precious magnesium provided in our diet. This leads to a magnesium deficiency and a host of health issues (see chapter 12).

Insulin also impacts the production of many anabolic hormones such as growth hormone, testosterone, and progesterone. These are hormones that are vital to both bone and muscle health. The insulin released in response to a bedtime snack will inhibit a needed nocturnal burst of growth hormone. As we increase insulin to cope with the refined sugars in our diet, we lose muscle mass and reduce bone building. Finally, insulin triggers cell growth which can help cancers grow. One of the strongest correlations in breast and colon cancers is the level of insulin. To protect against these cancers, we need to moderate the amount of insulin we secrete.

The most effective ways to moderate insulin secretion are to (1) avoid refined sugars in our diet, (2) avoid grazing, and (3) eat copious amounts of green vegetables. We need times during which we do not eat, do not trigger insulin release, and thus allow other hormones to do the vital work they are intended to do. We need plant compounds from green vegetables to help our bodies be more responsive to insulin.

CHAPTER SUMMARY

One of our goals on the TQI Diet is to free ourselves from insulin dominance and allow other metabolic hormones to play their intended roles and help maintain a healthy balance. To do this, we need to avoid grazing, eat more of the chlorophyll-containing parts of plants, and avoid non-nutritious foods that spike our blood sugar levels. This does not, however, mean that we should necessarily avoid foods that are high on the glycemic index. The glycemic index is only one factor in making healthy eating choices. Other factors include how rich the particular food is in antioxidants, essential fats, and other beneficial compounds.

CHAPTER TEN
Leptin Resistance

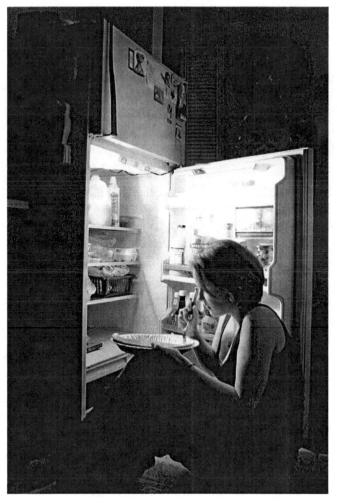

Bedtime snacks disrupt our leptin clocks.

Our fat cells use the hormone leptin to tell the brain how much energy is stored as fat at any given moment. When leptin levels are low—indicating less fat stored in the cells—the brain should increase our appetite, motivating us to replenish our energy stores. When leptin levels are high—indicating sufficient fat supplies—the brain should reduce our appetite. A properly functioning leptin system prevents us from gaining or losing too much weight by controlling and moderating our desire to eat.

If we eat the wrong foods and eat at the wrong time of the day, our leptin rhythm can be thrown off (see p. 39). If we constantly eat, we will constantly release bursts of leptin. Faced with a relentless barrage of leptin, the brain may stop responding to leptin. When the brain ignores leptin bursts, our desire to eat remains high, even though our body is flooded with leptin. This is referred to as leptin resistance. Leptin resistance, just like insulin resistance, increases abdominal fat and inflammation. It also can cause irresistible food cravings that sabotage our efforts to eat healthfully.

We can overcome leptin resistance by following five simple rules:

- Eat a breakfast rich in high-quality protein with fruits and vegetables, without grains, smoothies, or juices.

- Engage in some exercise, such as walking, between meals.

- Carefully avoid all sugar and refined grains.

- Do not graze between meals.

- Do not eat two to three hours (or longer) before bedtime.

CHAPTER ELEVEN

Calcium in the Diet

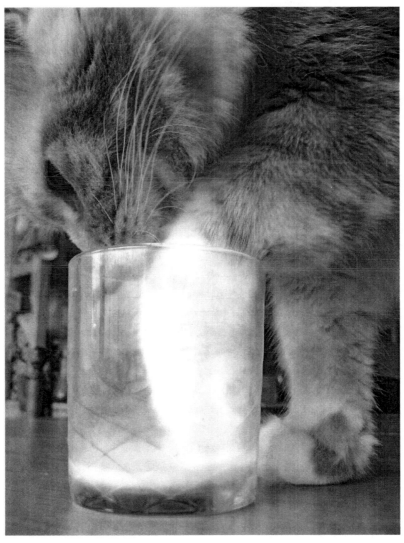

Dairy is not our only source of calcium.

We can lessen our exposure to environmental toxins by eating less (or no) dairy. But for the moment the prevailing medical opinion is that a post-menopausal woman should eat plenty of dairy and take a 1,200-1,500 mg calcium supplement each day to reduce her risk of osteoporosis. Giving up dairy raises the concern that we will not get enough calcium to maintain strong bones. Actually, dark leafy greens and many other foods are rich in calcium. For instance, three-fourths cup of collard greens provides more calcium than a glass of milk.[1] But it turns out the more important—and yet unanswered—question is: "How much calcium do we need?"

THREE STUDIES ON CALCIUM AND OSTEOPOROSIS

There are three interesting—and conflicting—studies that we will use to explore how our calcium intake affects our bone health:

The first study[2] is a review of existing studies correlating a woman's diet with the incidence of osteoporosis. Its conclusions were startling. A daily intake of 1,000 mg of calcium or more, whether through diet or supplement, did not prevent osteoporosis or vertebral fractures at all. That calcium did, however, increase the likelihood of hip fractures in some women by 64 percent. It is known that calcium will not increase bone strength if vitamin D levels are too low. So, the researchers attempted to determine if where a woman lived (and hence her vitamin D status) changed these results. It did not. Large amounts of calcium in the diet did not prevent, and sometimes worsened, osteoporosis.

---

[1] And, because greens feed our beneficial intestinal flora, we are better able to absorb the calcium in the collard greens.

[2] Bischoff-Ferrari HA, Dawson-Huges B, Baron JA, et al. Calcium intake and hip fracture risk in men & women. *Am J Clin Nutr* 2007; 86:1780-1790.

The second study[3] consisted of data from only 26 women. These women were osteoporotic, many with bone ratings below the fracture level on bone density tests. For six months, these women ate less protein, cut their intake of calcium in half (to 500 mg/day), and dramatically increased their daily intake of magnesium. At the end of the study, many of the women had moved above the fracture level, and their bones had improved dramatically. While these results are interesting, the number of people in the study is too small to have "statistical significance," and those same results might not show up in a larger study.

The third study[4] also reviewed many, but not all, of the existing studies correlating a woman's diet with the incidence of osteoporosis. It, however, reached the opposite conclusion to study number one: Women need to eat more protein and get more calcium in order to fend off osteoporosis.

We are all familiar with this chain of events. A study comes out suggesting we do something. Within a very short time, another study recommends that we do the exact opposite. Many people find it too difficult to sort through all of the conflicting information and basically give up. However, rather than give up, we might instead examine the funding for the opposing studies. Is there any potential bias involved?

Nutritional research foundations provided most of the funding for the first study. These groups have no financial interest in what people eat or what supplements they take. There was no apparent funding bias involved.

The second study failed to report on funding, presumably because it was a small pilot study.

The third study was connected to groups with a financial interest in how much protein and calcium people eat: Grants and

---

[3] Abraham GA, Grewal H. A total dietary program emphasizing magnesium rather than calcium. Effect on the mineral density of calcaneous bone in postmenopausal women on hormones. *J Repro Med* 1990; 35:503-507.

[4] Heaney RP, Layman DK. Amount and type of protein influences bone health. *Am J Clin Nutr* 2008; 87:1567S-1570S. See also Heaney RP. Calcium, dairy products and osteoporosis. *J Am Coll Nutr* 2000; 19:83S-99S.

paid speaking engagements were provided by the National Dairy Council, The Beefcheckoff, the National Cattlemen's Beef Association, and the Egg Nutrition Center.

Of course, the fact that funding (and other financial inducements) is provided by interest groups does not necessarily mean that the study's conclusions are invalid. However, funding is reported to provide transparency, because money can create a bias. In fact, one of the main problems with nutritional research in general is that so much of its funding comes from the food industry. The strikingly positive results achieved in the small second study ideally should be followed by a very large, properly designed follow-up study. If, in fact, we can reverse osteoporosis simply by eating less animal protein, cutting back on our calcium supplements, and eating food rich in magnesium (e.g., fish, green vegetables, nuts, and beans), we need to know that as soon as possible. At the same time, we cannot expect the National Dairy Council to fund a study that might end up recommending that we drink less milk and take less calcium; it would be contrary to its business interests.

Unfortunately, it will be decades before we know with certainty whether large amounts of calcium in the diet aggravate rather than prevent osteoporosis. Remember, it took decades to prove that smoking causes lung cancer. It took decades before cigarette ads were pulled off television and out of medical journals. It is taking decades to establish that bisphenol-A, a xenoestrogen, should not be in baby bottles. It is taking decades to determine whether hormone replacement therapy causes or prevents breast cancer, ovarian cancer, dementia, heart disease, etc. There are, however, increasing indications that we should avoid high doses of calcium. A New Zealand study looking at a dozen clinical trials involving some 12,000 patients found calcium supplementation to be associated with a 20% to 30% increase in heart attack risk. The lead researcher questioned the practice of supplementing with calcium in osteoporosis because calcium at best slightly reduces fracture risk but has a significant ability to cause heart attacks.[5]

---

[5]   Bolland MJ, Avenell A, Baron JA, et al. Effect of calcium supplements on

Chapter summary

There are two points of certainty when it comes to bone health: Adequate exercise and vitamin D are essential. We need to make sure that we engage in enough weight-bearing exercise (walking, running, etc.) and that we have adequate vitamin D levels if we wish to protect our bones. On other points, there is uncertainty.

The greater weight of scientific studies currently indicates that large amounts of dietary calcium are important for bone health. Increasingly, however, questions are being raised about the validity of those results. We have the review study finding that large amounts of calcium may not prevent osteoporosis, described above. We also have the study on calcium and heart health.

Questions are also raised by the following: (1) Our hunter/gatherer ancestors in general ate a diet low in calcium. Nonetheless, they did not appear to suffer from osteoporosis in regions where they ate a varied diet and got enough sunshine to make adequate amounts of vitamin D. (2) American women have been taking the recommended 1,200 to 1,500 mg of calcium/day and eating plenty of dairy for some time now, yet osteoporosis is on the rise, rather than on the decline. (3) Our magnesium intake is often too low. The U.S. recommended daily allowance (RDA) for magnesium is only 300 to 400 mg/day yet most Americans fail to get even that amount from their food. (4) Our current calcium recommendations are based on studies largely funded by interest groups.[6]

Thus, it is possible that the approach taken in the small Abraham study is correct: The best way to avoid osteoporosis is to eat less animal protein, less dairy, and more foods rich in magnesium (see chapter 16). It is also possible that current medical wisdom is correct: In order to avoid osteoporosis, you need to eat dairy daily, take a calcium and a vitamin D supplement, and get regular weight-bearing exercise. As an adult, you will have to make up

---

risk of myocardial infarction and cardiovascular events: meta-analysis. BMJ 341:doi:10.1136/bmj.c3691 (Published 29 July 2010).

[6] It has been reported that six out of seven of the review studies most frequently relied on to support current recommendations on calcium needs were funded by the dairy industry.

your own mind what to believe. But at least you now know that the current majority view on calcium supplementation may be incorrect.[7]

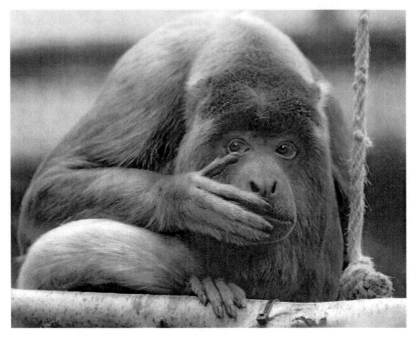

The studies on how much calcium we should take are contradictory and confusing.

---

[7] Not that long ago, conventional medical advice was to avoid taking vitamin D in excess of 600 to 800 units/day. Today, many people are taking 2,000 units (in some cases 50,000 units or more) per day on the advice of their physicians. Obviously, recommendations can change quickly and dramatically.

CHAPTER TWELVE

Magnesium's Many Roles

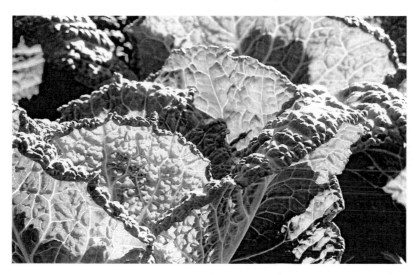

Dark, leafy greens are rich
in both magnesium and calcium.

Enzymes are biological catalysts that speed up chemical reactions and processes that would otherwise occur very slowly, if at all. Magnesium is a vital mineral because it regulates more than 300 of our enzymes, and many of those enzymes catalyze critical reactions. Magnesium helps maintain normal muscle and nerve function, keeps heart rhythm steady and bones strong. It plays a major role in energy metabolism and protein synthesis. As might be expected, magnesium deficiency contributes to a wide array of ailments because of its central role in so many important functions.

RELAXING MUSCLE CONTRACTIONS

Magnesium is essential because it relaxes our muscles. We use calcium and magnesium ions alternately to contract and relax muscle fibers. During contraction, muscle cells are flooded with calcium. Muscles relax when magnesium instead concentrates in the cell. A lack of magnesium leaves muscles throughout the body vulnerable to excessive contraction.[1] A magnesium deficiency can cause painful calf and foot cramps but magnesium also affects muscle layers around our blood vessels and muscles in other organs. As muscles contract around smaller blood vessels, individuals with Raynaud's syndrome experience pain and numbness. Painful cramping of the uterine muscle during menses (dymenorrhea) increases if magnesium is deficient. In asthmatics, magnesium deficiency increases the frequency of bronchial spasms as the muscles around the bronchi constrict.

REGULATING BLOOD PRESSURE

Another of magnesium's major roles is to regulate blood pres-

---

[1] This deficiency may be "real," in other words there is simply not enough magnesium in the system. Or it may be "relative," in other words there is too much calcium relative to the amount of magnesium present.

sure and maintain a healthy circulatory system. The Joint National Committee on High Blood Pressure urges us to get enough magnesium in our diet in order to prevent high blood pressure. If we are deficient in magnesium, muscles around our major blood vessels contract, raising blood pressure.

REGULATING BLOOD FATS

The liver needs magnesium to maintain an appropriate level of cholesterol in our blood. A lack of magnesium raises triglyceride levels and lowers HDL, the good cholesterol.[2]

REGULATING HEART RHYTHMS

Magnesium is needed for proper functioning of the heart muscle as well. Low body stores of magnesium increase the risk of abnormal heart rhythms, which are associated with both heart attacks and strokes. Individuals with higher levels of magnesium have a lower risk of coronary heart disease.

REGULATING BONE HEALTH

Magnesium is important for bone health, as indicated by the Abraham osteoporosis study (see chapter 11).

REGULATING BLOOD SUGAR LEVELS

Magnesium also influences the release and activity of insulin. When our blood sugar levels are too high, we start losing magnesium in the urine. That is why individuals with poorly controlled diabetes usually have low blood levels of magnesium. Lack of magnesium is also causative in insulin resistance or syndrome X and in weight gain.

GOOD SOURCES OF MAGNESIUM

Our primary source needs to be our food because it appears that magnesium must come from food to be fully functional in our bodies: Studies show that dietary magnesium lowered blood pressure; magnesium supplements did not. Our best sources of magnesium are plant foods such as nuts, whole grains, legumes, and

---

[2] Sugars deplete magnesium stores in the liver. This is one reason why excess sugars in the diet tend to raise our cholesterol levels.

vegetables. Some drinking waters, in areas where the water is hard, are a good source. Fish and other animal foods also provide higher amounts of magnesium but based on the amount of magnesium per calorie, plants are the most impressive source. Plants contain

Food, amount	Magnesium (in mg)
Pumpkin and squash seed kernels, roasted, 1 oz	151
Swiss chard, 1 cup cooked	150
Brazil nuts, 1 oz	107
Halibut, cooked, 3 oz	91
Quinoa, dry, 1/4 cup	89
Spinach, canned, 1/2 cup	81
Almonds, 1 oz	78
Spinach, fresh cooked, 1/2 cup	78
Cashews, 1 oz	74
Soybeans, cooked, 1/2 cup	74
Pine nuts, dried, 1 oz	71
White beans, canned, 1/2 cup	67
Black beans, cooked, 1/2 cup	60
Bulgur, dry, 1/4 cup	57
Artichoke hearts, cooked, 1/2 cup	50
Lima beans, baby, 1/2 cup	50
Beet greens, cooked, 1/2 cup	49
Navy beans, cooked 1/2 cup	48
Tofu, firm made with nigari, 1/2 cup	47
Okra, 1/2 cup	47
Hazelnuts, 1 oz	46
Brown rice, cooked 1/2 cup	42
Collards, boiled, 1 cup	38
Broccoli, cooked, 1 cup	33

magnesium because magnesium is at the heart of the chlorophyll molecule they use to harvest sunshine. Magnesium is abundant in the parts of plants that harvest sunshine but it is also stored in seeds and nuts for the use of future generations of plants.

EVENTS THAT DEPLETE MAGNESIUM

Unfortunately, most of us do not get the recommended daily allowance of magnesium (300 to 400 mg/day). Moreover, we compound the problem by doing many things that deplete our magnesium stores:

✳ We eat refined grains instead of whole grains. When flour is refined and processed, the magnesium-rich germ and bran are removed.

✳ We drink alcohol. Alcohol is a magnesium diuretic that causes a substantial loss of magnesium in the urine. Chronic drinking depletes body stores of magnesium. Many of the adverse effects of alcoholism are attributed to the resulting magnesium deficiency. Alcohol's effect on magnesium may be the reason why a daily glass of wine increased the incidence of heart arrhythmias in women in one study. In addition, while the liver is detoxifying the alcohol we drink, it stops converting glycogen to glucose, and blood sugar levels tend to plummet. This increases our cravings for sugary, refined grain treats that further deplete our magnesium stores.

✳ We often ingest relatively too much calcium compared to the amount of magnesium in our diet. High levels of calcium block magnesium absorption. This is what is at the core of the ongoing debate on the wisdom of recommending large amounts of dairy and calcium supplements as a treatment for osteoporosis (see chapter 11).

✳ We eat simple sugars, refined carbohydrates, white flour, white rice, and high-fructose corn syrup. Magnesium-deficient rats fed a diet high in refined grains and sugars had much higher levels of triglycerides as well as higher LDL ("bad" cholesterol) with lowered HDL ("good" cholesterol). The combination of low magnesium and high sugar intake also increases insulin resistance.

The fructose added to our food aggravates further.[1] Free fructose interferes with the heart's use of magnesium, leading to an increased tendency to form blood clots that can cause stroke and heart attacks.

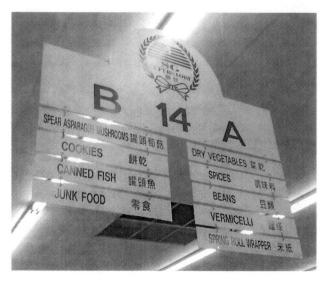

Preserve healthy magnesium levels by
avoiding the junk food aisle at the grocery store

✻ We take diuretics to control our blood pressure. Diuretics—even potassium-sparing diuretics—do not spare magnesium. It is noteworthy that the elderly (who tend to be low in magnesium due to poor diet) often use diuretics to control blood pressure. The increased magnesium deficiency may then increase their risk of stroke and heart arrhythmias. Remember, taking magnesium supplements to control blood pressure is not as effective as increasing the magnesium in your food.

---

[1] The problem is not caused by the fructose in the fruit we eat but rather is due to the amount of fructose added to other foods. In 1980 the average person in the U.S. ate 39 pounds of fructose and 84 pounds of white sugar. In 1994 the average person ate 83 pounds of fructose and 66 pounds of sugar, providing 19 percent of total calories. Today approximately 25 percent of our total calories typically comes from sugars, with the larger portion as fructose.

✱ Our blood sugar tends to run high, which depletes magnesium stores in the liver. Insulin also causes a loss of magnesium whether taken as a drug or secreted by the pancreas to deal with blood sugar spikes.

✱ We drink sodas; they too deplete magnesium in the body.

✱ Other causes of magnesium loss include chronic pain, coffee, diarrhea, and many intestinal disorders, too much exercise, high salt intake, and stress.

CHAPTER SUMMARY

Eating a more wholesome diet, rich in magnesium, and limiting foods that deplete magnesium often has an immediate and positive effect on our health. The proportionate meal provides a simple and easy way to accomplish this goal.

CHAPTER THIRTEEN
Chocolate

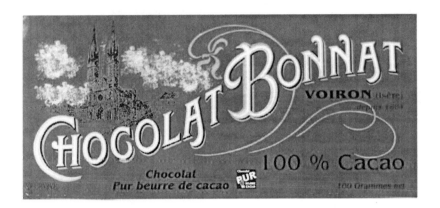

You may eat all the unsweetened 100% chocolate you wish during the Elimination Phase. Once past the Elimination and Testing Phases, you may also eat one or two squares of sweetened, 75% or darker chocolate a day.[1]

Chocolate comes from the cocoa bean, a tropical fruit rich in interesting antioxidants and plant fats that have a very beneficial effect on the circulatory system. For instance, a group of Harvard doctors studied the health and diet of a Caribbean tribe that cooked with cocoa beans and also drank on average five cups of hot chocolate made with water rather than milk each day. Tribal members had no age-related hypertension whatsoever when following their traditional diet. However, once they moved to the city and stopped drinking many cups of cocoa a day, they began developing hypertension. In other words, their traditional diet with its many cups of daily water-based cocoa maintained normal blood pressure. The antioxidants in chocolate prevent fats from clogging their arteries. These compounds also slow blood clotting and reduce the risk of heart attacks and stroke. They may increase insulin sensitivity as well.

Despite these potential health benefits, chocolate still carries the stigma that it may trigger migraines, contains too much caffeine, causes acne outbreaks, and/or is a common cause of food sensitivities. First, the chocolate-migraine connection is unclear. Chocolate may trigger migraines in some but certainly is not a cause in all migraine sufferers. So, if you suffer from migraines you should test to see if it aggravates your headaches; it may not.

---

[1] The percentage tells how much chocolate is in the bar. In a 75% bar, 75% is chocolate and 25% consists of sweeteners and emulsifiers. The oxidative stress that one or two squares of sweetened 75% chocolate causes is offset by the antioxidants in the chocolate itself. If you eat more, the problems from the sugars begin to predominate and cause problems.

Others worry about the caffeine in chocolate. In fact, chocolate contains only negligible amounts of caffeine. Instead, it contains theobromine, a compound related to caffeine. Theobromine is a much gentler stimulant than caffeine—of course, you may still find it overstimulating and something you wish to avoid.

Chocolate is also often said to cause acne but studies have failed to confirm that chocolate consistently triggers acne outbreaks. A more likely cause of acne is the milk often combined with chocolate: Women drinking three or more glasses of milk a day are significantly more likely to have severe acne.

Chocolate rarely causes true allergies or sensitivities. Often the reaction blamed on the chocolate instead is due to nuts or soy (often in the form of soy lecithin) present in the chocolate bar. Nonetheless, chocolate may be a trigger food for you. If you suspect that you are sensitive to chocolate, you should eliminate it and then reintroduce it during the Testing Phase using the protocol for wheat (see chapter 22).

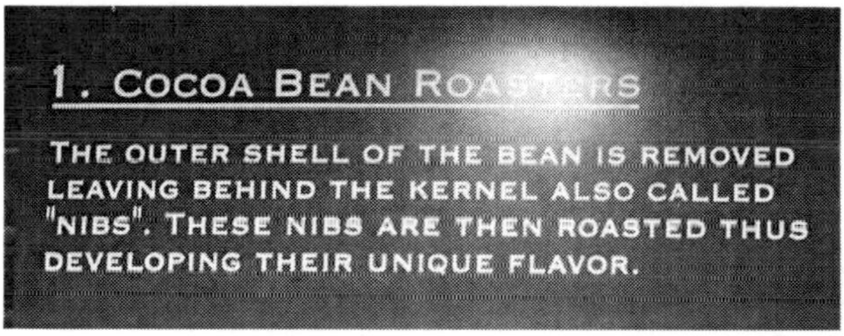

1. COCOA BEAN ROASTERS

THE OUTER SHELL OF THE BEAN IS REMOVED LEAVING BEHIND THE KERNEL ALSO CALLED "NIBS". THESE NIBS ARE THEN ROASTED THUS DEVELOPING THEIR UNIQUE FLAVOR.

Cocoa nibs are bitter and gritty eaten alone
but are tasty when eaten with ripe fruits.

CHAPTER SUMMARY

Unsweetened chocolate, rich in antioxidants that are especially beneficial to the circulatory system, is treated as a vegetable. It may be eaten freely as long as it is unsweetened.

CHAPTER FOURTEEN

Calories

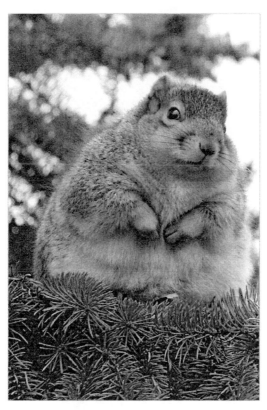

Whether we gain or lose weight
involves more than the calories we eat

Current wisdom is that whether we gain or lose weight is determined entirely by our calorie intake. If we eat more calories than we burn, we gain weight. If we eat less, we lose weight. What we eat is said to have no effect; it is only the total calories consumed that matter. We are also told that it does not matter when we eat or under what conditions we eat.

However, the calorie approach to weight loss and weight gain is not entirely accurate. Instead, what we eat, when we eat, and the conditions under which we eat change how our bodies process calories. This means that the calorie-in, calorie-out approach to weight loss is not as helpful as currently thought.

The following studies were done on animals, not humans, but animals are used in research because the results are supposed to reflect what happens in humans. These studies show that:

- Animals subjected to stress gain weight, even when they exercise more and eat less than non-stressed animals.

- Animals fed fast food gain more weight than animals eating the same number of calories from the "normal" diet for their species.

- Animals stressed and fed fast food gain more weight than stressed animals fed healthier food. They gain more weight than non-stressed animals eating fast food even though all animals ate the same number of calories.

- Nocturnal animals (who eat at night and sleep during the day) gain more weight if they are fed in the daytime rather than at night even though all animals in the study ate the same number of calories.

What this means is that:

- ❧ Our biochemistry changes when we are under stress and we process calories differently. Most of us gain weight under stressful circumstances just as the lab rats did.

- ❧ Our biochemistry changes when we eat poorly and fail to get needed nutrients. A poor diet predisposes most of us to gain weight even when we are watching our calories carefully.

- ❧ Our biochemistry changes over a 24-hour day. We are not nocturnal and we process calories differently when we eat late at night rather than during the day.

CHAPTER SUMMARY

When we eat healthy foods, do not eat late at night, and reduce our stress levels, we can lose weight even though we still are eating the same number of calories as when we ate poorly, late at night, and were under substantial stress.

Of course, calories matter. We do not need to count them, however, as long as we eat properly. First, we do not usually overeat healthy foods. Second, when we consistently eat nutritious foods, our appetite stabilizes. Part of the reason we overeat bad foods is because we must eat a greater quantity as we try to satisfy our need for nutrients from foods that are nutrient poor.

The stress/weight gain studies also are important for another reason: Bad foods are much more harder on us when we are stressed. To avoid this negative effect, we should make sure that we are in a good mood and in good company when we eat poorly. If we are attending a dysfunctional family gathering, or a stress-filled business dinner, we need to avoid inflammatory foods because they are much harder on us—and more fattening—than they would be under other circumstances. Of course, we all also need to work on reducing stress in all of its many forms.

CHAPTER FIFTEEN

Stress

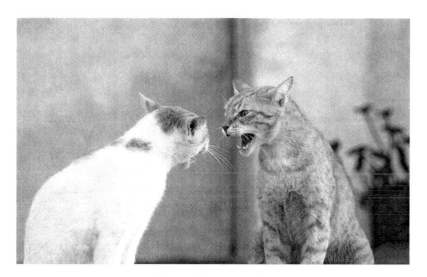

Stressful encounter

Our bodies must be able to respond quickly to physical stress, the classic example being running away from a tiger. In response to stress, our adrenals release adrenalin and cortisol. These hormones increase our heart rate and blood sugar levels and decrease "non-essential" functions (such as digestion) to enable us to take off running and not run out of steam. We use this same hormonal response for any type of emotional or physical stress (such as a disease). If we are constantly under stress, our hormones end up out of balance and our bodies begin to malfunction.

Persistent stress disrupts the daily rhythm of many different hormones. For instance, cortisol should rise in the morning to give us energy to start our day. It should fall at night while growth hormone and melatonin increase. An upset in this rhythm can lead to "night-eating syndrome" and a decreased appetite in the morning. Sleep deprivation, another common occurrence in stress, increases grehlin (the "hunger hormone") and decreases leptin (the "satiety hormone"). Women under stress have higher levels of cortisol, more fat accumulated around their bellies, higher levels of cholesterol, and lower levels of testosterone and thyroid hormone. Lower testosterone levels can lead to muscle loss and fat accumulation. Growth hormone and HDL also drop.

The bottom line is that we put on intra-abdominal fat when we are stressed. In turn, this internal fat is a form of physical stress that increases the release of stress hormones. The increase in stress hormones leads to more fat storage, and on and on. The stress hormones throw our digestive hormones out of balance and we are more inclined to make poor food choices. Eating poorly while under stress changes how we process calories, enhancing abdominal weight gain and inflammation. Chronic stress leads us into a negative, downward spiral. Eating well breaks the downward spiral but we also need to work on reducing stress so that we can move into a positive, upward spiral toward health.

WAYS TO REDUCE STRESS

1. IDENTIFY AND REDUCE CAUSES OF STRESS

The first step in reducing stress is to fully understand the stress you are under. Make a list of physical stressors (being overweight, a chronic illness, toxins, sugar, high-fructose corn syrup, saturated fats, alcohol, tobacco, drugs). Then add the psychological stressors (depression, family responsibilities, anxiety, low self-esteem, state of the world, financial worries). Over time, work on reducing them and improve how you cope with those you cannot reduce.

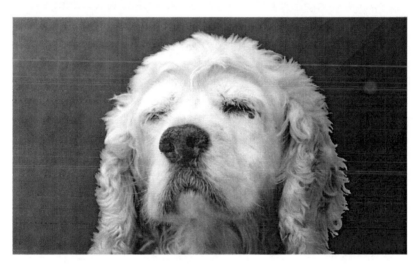

Meditation is calming

2. PRACTICE CALMING DOWN

There are many activities that make us less reactive to stress: Meditation, prayer, yoga, Qi gong, Jin Shin Jyutsu, massage, dance, etc. all reduce stress. Try some of them and find one that works for you.

3. TAKE SAUNAS, STEAM BATHS, HOT BATHS

Soaking in hot water or sweating helps us relax because it speeds up the processing of our stress hormones. A hot bath or a soak in a hot tub relaxes muscle tension and reduces our stress level.

4. EXERCISE

Our bodies are designed to move and exercise helps restore our hormonal rhythms. We function better when we move. Walk, swim, garden, bicycle, or take an exercise class.

5. EAT FOODS THAT PREVENT STRESS DAMAGE

We are better able to ward off the damaging effects of stress when we eat properly. We need dark leafy greens, fruits, vegetables, nuts, and whole grains to help us cope with stress. Consider whether you need an omega-3 supplement such as fish oil or flax seed.

6. USE ADAPTOGENIC HERBS

Adaptogenic herbs are used to make us less reactive to stress. When we are less reactive, we are better able to, for instance, endure a traffic jam without losing our temper. Adaptogens typically are taken daily and slowly, over time, help quiet our stress response. They include eleuthero or Siberian ginseng (*Eleutherococcus senticosus*), rhodiola (*Rhodiola rosea*), ashwagandha (*Withania somniferum*), American ginseng (*Panax quinquefolius*), Chinese ginseng (*Panax ginseng*), and schisandra (*Schisandra chinensis*). Most can be taken either as teas, capsules, or tinctures. Ask a health care provider trained in botanical medicine if an adaptogen might benefit you.

7. EXPERIENCE HOW COMFORT FOODS INCREASE STRESS

Under stress, most of us reach for "comfort foods," foods that usually are high in simple carbohydrates and poor quality fats. Studies show that our comfort foods actually temporarily reduce our stress hormones. They do make us feel better. We have subconsciously internalized this and some part of us "knows" that a cookie will make us feel less stressed. This is part of the reason we are drawn to the "wrong" foods under stress.

Unfortunately, this relief only lasts for a moment. As we secrete insulin in response to our sugary snack, the insulin raises our stress hormone levels higher than they were before the snack. Soon, very soon, we feel worse than we did before we ate our comfort food. However, we do not fully understand that our comfort food is making us feel worse. Instead, we blame the resulting "bad" feelings on our lack of willpower. Our failure to fully understand our desire to "self-medicate" against stress with comfort foods often leads us to abandon healthy eating: We have a strong desire to alleviate stress with the wrong foods, we stress out over our lack of willpower, and then give up altogether.

Instead, take a different approach. When you become stressed and tempted to eat an inflammatory food, first observe yourself. What foods are you craving? What does your yearning reflect about the underlying attitude giving rise to your desire? (See the study on the following page.) Wait a few minutes, move, and breathe. If you cannot resist, then choose the comfort food you really desire. Notice how the food momentarily makes you feel better. Then, when inevitably you feel worse, remember that it is the effect of the inflammatory food you ate that is making you feel poorly. Begin to associate inflammatory foods with their negative effects. Quit blaming your lack of willpower.

Also, before you give in and eat your comfort food, make a sincere commitment to soon do something good for your body. Whether you are in the mood or not, promise to eat some vegetables soon: Make a salad, some vegetable soup, or heat up some frozen vegetables. It does not matter that the dish is not enticing and that you do not want vegetables. Eat them because their antioxidants will help quiet the oxidative stress and will break the desire to have yet more of the wrong food. Then let go of the episode and simply return to eating properly. Over time, following this plan of action—especially making yourself eat compensatory vegetables—will break the cycle of using inflammatory foods in a vain attempt to self-medicate stress with comfort foods.

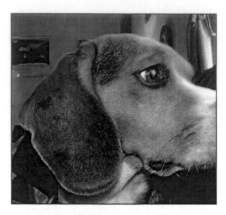

My Person is Leaving Me Alone...

MOODS AND COMFORT FOODS

There is a small but interesting study that looked at how different moods and states of mind affected which comfort foods people ate. The volunteers in the study were offered a buffet of various foods after filling out a questionnaire that revealed their mood.

This study found:

- People with anger issues preferred meats or hard, crunchy foods.

- People struggling with depression chose sweets and sugars.

- People feeling lonely preferred starchy foods such as pasta and bread.

- People struggling with anxiety went for soft, sweet foods such as custard and ice cream.

- People feeling overwhelmed by stress preferred salty foods.

- People with jealousy issues showed no preference; they ate any and all of the foods offered.

CHAPTER SIXTEEN

Protein in the Diet

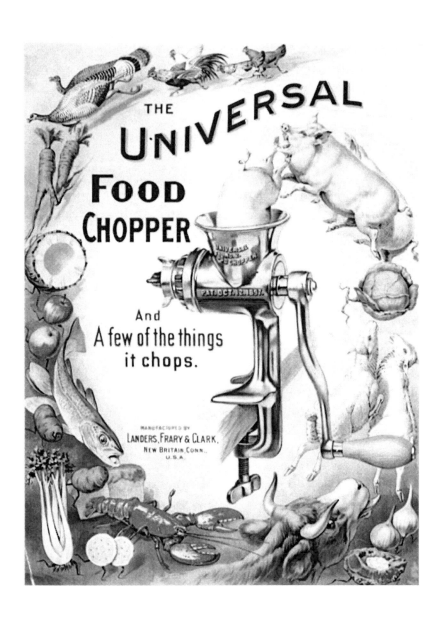

Americans are a bit obsessed with protein. Many who regularly eat animal products nonetheless worry about whether they have adequate protein to maintain lean muscle. Many feel that they need a protein shake to start the day and a protein bar pick-me-up mid-afternoon. Frequently, we blame fatigue and lethargy on a need for more meat in the diet. In fact, our protein needs are easily met by almost any diet.

WHAT ARE PROTEINS?

Proteins are made up of different combinations of compounds called amino acids. We make some 50,000 different proteins and they are critical to our health and survival. Hemoglobin that carries oxygen from our lungs to our cells is a protein. Insulin, the hormone that helps maintain our blood sugar levels, is a protein. Our digestive enzymes are proteins, as are all of the other enzymes that enable us to function.

The body makes proteins by joining various amino acids together in long chains that fold into a three-dimensional shape. This shape is critical for protein function. We use 22 different amino acids to make the many different proteins we need, and we can make most of those amino acids from scratch. However, we cannot make 8 or 9 of the amino acids needed to build proteins. These amino acids are called essential amino acids because we must get them in the food we eat.[1]

ANIMAL PRODUCTS ARE COMPLETE PROTEINS

Foods that contain the "right" balance of all of the essential amino acids we need are called *complete proteins*. All animal foods are complete proteins. Quinoa is also a complete protein. Other

---

[1] The essential amino acids are threonine, valine, methionine, leucine, isoleucine, phenylalanine, tryptophan, and histidine (some histidine synthesis is possible in adults but not children).

foods also have all eight essential amino acids but not in the exact ratio we need. Each has its own ratio of the essential amino acids. If we do not eat complete proteins, we must either eat very large amounts of a single incomplete food[2] or eat a variety of different foods to get all the essential amino acids we need.

Many people worry about getting their essential amino acids if they are not eating animal proteins. Much of this concern derives from a book published in the 1970s, *Diet for a Small Planet.* This book encouraged people to switch to a plant-based diet but cautioned that those who eliminated animal products would have to carefully combine foods at every meal. For instance, if rice were served for lunch, beans would have to be added to achieve a balance of essential amino acids. Fortunately, such protein combining is *not* necessary.

We now know that we "pool" the amino acids from our food and maintain a supply of essential amino acids sufficient to satisfy our protein-building needs for at least 24 hours (and probably 48 hours). We need not worry about getting all of our essential amino acids from each meal. As long as we eat a variety of foods over the course of each day, we will get all of the essential amino acids that we need. We may have beans for breakfast and rice for dinner rather than combining them in one meal. We can safely ignore whether our proteins are complete or incomplete—provided we eat a variety of foods over the course of a day. On this plan, we eat a wide variety of leafy greens, colorful fruits and vegetables, and high-quality proteins. This ensures a full complement of essential amino acids even if we do not eat animal products.

How much protein do we need?

Adults need 20 to 30 grams of protein daily (grams/day) according to the World Health Organization (WHO). The U.S. recommends slightly over twice that amount, 45 to 70 grams/day.

---

[2] Incomplete foods are not lacking in any of the essential amino acids; they instead contain low amounts of some. If you ate enough potatoes (6 to 8 per day), you would get all your essential amino acids. However, a diet of only potatoes would not have all of the other nutrients you need and would not be healthy.

Except in starvation,[3] diets around the world equal or exceed the U.S. recommendations:

Hardworking farmers in rural Asian societies, engaged in large amounts of physical activity, typically get about 40 to 75 grams daily, eating rice with vegetables and very little animal protein. Individuals on a vegan diet, diets without animal proteins of any kind, average 35 to 75 grams/day. The Western diet, rich in meat, dairy, eggs, beans, and nuts, on average provides about 100 to 160 grams/day, or often about five times more protein than recommended by WHO. A traditional Eskimo, eating marine animals, or someone on the Atkins diet might be consuming 200 to 350 grams a day—more than ten times the necessary amount.

Diet	Protein in Diet
World Health Org Recommends	20-30 grams/day
U.S. Recommends	45-70 grams/day
Traditional Asian Diet	40-75 grams/day
McDougall Diet (Vegan)	35-75 grams/day
Average Western Diet	75-160 grams/day
Zone Diet provides	160 grams/day
South Beach Diet	100-250 grams/day
Atkins Diet	150-350 grams/day

Many Americans worry unless they eat animal proteins every day, if not at every meal. Then, just to be on the safe side, many have a daily protein shake that may add another 40 to 50 grams of protein, in the belief the shake is needed to maintain muscle strength, overcome weakness, and avert fatigue. There are always a few students taking my classes who proclaim that they are feeling weak and tired, and need more protein (usually as dairy and beef) to maintain their vigor on the Elimination Phase. In fact, the weakness and fatigue some experience initially happens

---

[3]   Protein deficiency may also be a problem in people with eating disorders, in those on low-calorie diets, in the seriously ill, or in the elderly who no longer are able to shop and care for themselves properly.

when we eat too few calories or our meals and snacks are too light (see p. 135).

There is a small nugget of truth buried in our worry about protein since we must eat protein daily in order to be able to make and repair our own proteins. We lose about three grams of protein daily as we shed skin and slough off intestinal lining. We also repair muscle and other damaged proteins. Nonetheless, the fact remains that, except in starvation, we easily get what we need because all foods contain protein. For instance, every half-cup of vegetables provides two grams of protein, every half-cup of fruit provides one gram. Beans, nuts, and seeds provide more concentrated amounts. If we eat chicken, fish, and eggs we add significantly more protein.[4] We need not worry about getting enough protein. Unless we are ill, we do not need protein supplements. Our problem is not getting enough protein; rather, the problem is that we usually get too much.

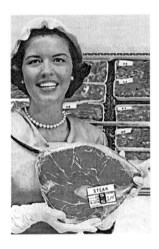

PROBLEMS WITH EXCESS PROTEIN
EXCESS PROTEIN BURDENS THE LIVER AND KIDNEYS

We need to consider what happens to excess protein because most of us eat protein beyond our needs. Whenever we eat more of something than we need, our body has two options: It can store the excess or it can excrete it.

---

[4] An ounce of almonds or cashews provides about 7 grams of protein. An egg provides about 6 grams, a half-cup of soybeans about 15 grams, 3 ounces of fish about 22 grams, 3.5 ounces of chicken about 30 grams.

The body does not store excess protein.[5] Instead, it is broken down and excreted (removed from the body). The excess is processed in the liver where it is broken down into acidic waste products. This waste includes compounds such as ammonia that damage the liver. The acidic waste is then shipped to the kidneys and eliminated in the urine. The acidic waste also damages the kidneys as it transits through them. This damage is cumulative and builds over time: On average a person on a Western high-protein diet loses 25% of kidney function by age 70, mostly due to the acid waste caused by eating too much protein.

A common treatment for people (or aging cats) with early kidney problems is a low-protein diet. People in liver failure are also often placed on low-protein diets. In advanced liver failure, patients often fall into a coma from the build-up of protein breakdown products (hepatic coma). Low protein diets are used because cutting protein reduces the burden on stressed livers and kidneys. Finally, excess protein is also associated with gout and kidney stones. An ounce of prevention is worth a pound of cure: There are sound reasons to avoid protein excesses.

EXCESS PROTEIN CONTRIBUTES TO OSTEOPOROSIS

Excess protein is also a factor in osteoporosis.[6] Worldwide, rates of hip fractures increase in step with the consumption of animal protein. People from the U.S., Canada, Norway, Sweden, Australia, and New Zealand have the highest intake of animal proteins. They also have the highest rates of osteoporosis. The lowest rates of osteoporosis are among peoples who eat the least animal product—people from rural Asia and Africa on traditional diets (these peoples also consume less calcium). Unfortunately, as Asia has adopted a more Western diet, higher in animal proteins, osteoporosis rates there have begun to climb dramatically.

---

[5]   If we could, excess protein would be stored as muscle and the average American would look like a body builder. A quick look around will confirm that that is not happening.

[6]   This is hotly contested by the dairy industry, while other academic scientists say that the link between excess animal protein and osteoporosis is as well established as that between smoking and lung cancer.

If you would like to calculate your personal protein needs, and determine at what point your intake becomes excessive, go to http://www.indoorclimbing.com.

Meat, poultry, fish, seafood, and hard cheeses are highly acidic foods. As the liver breaks down amino acids from these foods, acidic waste products are generated that must be shipped to the kidneys for excretion. These waste products travel from the liver to our kidneys in our blood. Our blood pH, however, must be kept in a very narrow range and we have to buffer acidic waste dumped into the bloodstream. Carbonate, citrate, and sodium are released from the bones to neutralize the acid, and in the process, calcium is leached out with them. The kidneys attempt to recapture the calcium but the sulfur-containing amino acids in the animal foods interfere. As a result, calcium is lost in the urine. Doubling animal protein intake increases the loss of calcium by 50%. Ultimately, excess animal protein increases daily urinary calcium loss. In contrast, fruit and vegetable proteins have an alkaline effect, and help preserve bones. (See table on p. 178.)

EXCESS PROTEIN ELEVATES CORTISOL LEVELS

The acidity resulting from a diet high in animal proteins also raises cortisol levels. Cortisol is a natural steroid hormone associated with our fight-or-flight response to stress. Elevated cortisol contributes to rapid bone loss—just as taking steroid medication for arthritis causes severe osteoporosis. So, a combination of stress and a diet high in dairy and other animal products contributes significantly to the rising rate of osteoporosis.

CHAPTER SUMMARY

The proportionate meal helps counteract the effect of animal proteins. First, we no longer make protein the centerpiece of our meals which helps us avoid excess proteins. Second, we always combine protein with twice as much fruits and vegetables so that their alkalizing effect may counter the negative, acidic effect animal proteins have on our liver, kidneys, and bone.

Acid Load Placed on Kidneys per 100 calories	
Cheddar cheese	10.0
Fish (cod)	9.3
Chicken	7.0
Beef	6.3
Peas	1.0
Wheat flour	1.0
Banana	-6.0
Potato	-5.0
Apple	-5.0
Tomatoes	-18.0
Spinach	-56.0

A positive number shows an acidic effect; a negative number shows an alkaline, non-damaging effect.

The conclusion that excess animal protein is a cause of osteoporosis typically is based on epidemiological studies. These studies have shown that the highest rates of osteoporosis occur in the Northern hemisphere where people eat the most animal protein. Historically, Asia had low rates of osteoporosis, even though Asian women often are very fine boned. However, as Asia has adopted the Western diet high in animal proteins, osteoporosis has become rampant.

According to The China Study,[1] excess animal protein in the diet is also associated with high rates of cancer and cardiovascular disease. The China Study makes a strong case that we would be healthier if we did not eat animal protein at all, a highly controversial concept in the United States.

---

[1] Campbell TC, Campbell TM. *The China Study.* Dallas, TX: Benbella Books, 2006.

CHAPTER SEVENTEEN
Quality of Animal Products

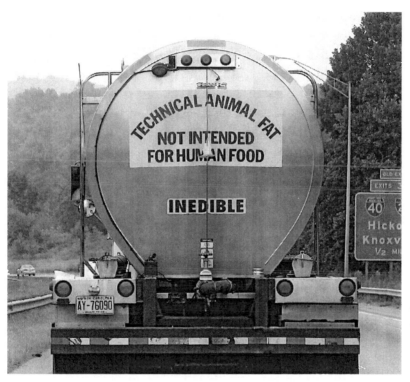

Strange foods travel our highways

During the Elimination Phase, we eat a limited variety of animal products. During the Testing Phase, we eat dairy for three days. Once the Testing Phase is complete, we shape a long-term eating plan that suits our individual needs and food preferences. For many, this means eating both dairy and a variety of other animal products. We may choose to eat lean cuts of various meats on a regular basis and any other meats as "special-occasion" foods. But, as we add these foods back into our diet, it is important to make "quality choices" if we are to maintain our health.

ANIMALS ARE WHAT THEY EAT

Chickens leading normal lives eat weeds, seeds, and insects, and lay eggs with a healthy ratio of essential fats (see chapter 6). Unfortunately, most chickens are confined and fed a different diet. Their eggs usually have an omega-6:3 ratio that is far from ideal because their diet is low in omega-3s.

Most conventional food animals are not fed the ideal diet for their species. Instead, they are usually fed a diet containing grease, bone meal, and byproducts made from rendered euthanized pets, road kill, dead farm animals, manure, and supermarket rejects (meats, poultry, and fish that did not sell by their expiration date). These unsavory items are heated, cooked, and pressed into various grain-based feed products and fed to chickens, cows, and virtually all food animals.

Flea collars from euthanized pets are not removed in the rendering process. The insecticide patches are left on dead farm animals. No one removes the plastic wrapping or the styrofoam containers holding the rotting supermarket rejects. Rendered products also include a certain amount of rocks, gravel, dirt, and cattle, pig, and poultry manure. This "food" may contain drugs and hormones that are not destroyed in the rendering process.

Sodium phenobarbital used to euthanize pets passes unchanged into the final products. Most likely other chemicals and toxins do as well.

One resulting rendering product is "technical animal fat." Federal regulations require that trucks or trains hauling technical animal fat label their tankers with 11-inch tall lettering reading: "Technical Animal Fat. Not intended for human food. Inedible." So, where does all of the inedible animal fat go? It is fed to animals that we later eat.[1]

This feed, along with genetically modified corn or soy, is fed to animals crammed into tiny, confined spaces. The poor living conditions combined with the poor-quality feed stresses the animals and makes them vulnerable to infections and disease. To overcome their vulnerability, they are often treated prophylactically with antibiotics and other drugs to enable them to survive until slaughter. Animals are also fed antibiotics to promote faster growth. Each year an estimated 13.5 million pounds of antibiotics—the same classes of drugs used in human medicine—are routinely added to animal feed or water. Some of the animal drugs contain arsenic, a known carcinogen, and arsenic ends up in meat from animals fed these drugs.[2]

The food we eat is increasingly dangerous to our health because of the poor quality of the feed and living conditions of our food animals. Once upon a time—and not all that long ago—people made eggnog from raw egg yolks, a practice now condemned by the FDA as entirely too dangerous. Children once licked the bowls while the homemade cookies baked. Nestle's refrigerated chocolate chip cookie dough was recalled at one point when people suffered serious *E. coli* infections after eating the raw cookie dough. In response, Nestle's website told us: We should not eat anything containing raw eggs even if the eggs in the cookie dough have been pasteurized!

---

[1] For instance, a chicken feed ad urges chicken farmers to buy their "high-quality technical animal fat" because it will increase the weight of the hens and cause them to lay larger eggs—at much lower cost than other feed.

[2] We are also exposed to arsenic in our water supply contaminated by runoff from factory farms.

Today, most supermarket chickens carry pathogenic microbes such as salmonella and campylobacter. Health officials advise us we must cook our chicken fully and scrub any surface that comes in contact with it very well with hot, soapy water. In fact, it is recommended that we have dedicated cutting boards for our poultry or meats. In a recent study, 70% of pork samples tested positive for MRSA (multidrug-resistant *Staphylococcus aureus*). Beef recalls are more and more frequent. We are warned never to eat hamburgers cooked rare because the meat so frequently is contaminated with pathogenic microbes.

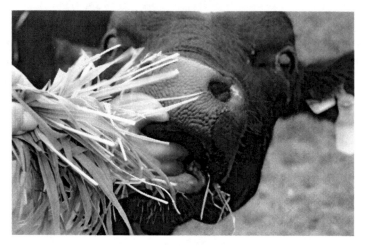

Cows thrive on grass

Cattle are natural grass eaters. Their digestive systems cannot handle a corn diet. Corn causes health problems for cows, including liver abscesses that increase the need for antibiotics and other drugs. Recalls of food contaminated with the kidney-destroying pathogen *E. coli* O157:H7 would be infrequent if cattle were raised properly. Finally, pesticide tolerances for animal feed are higher than for human food, and animal products are a source of persistent pesticides and insecticides (see chapter 8). Wild fish eating their natural diet of phytoplankton are a rich source of omega-3 fats. Farmed fish fed byproducts and manure are instead rich in omega-6 fats and much, much higher in toxins such as flame retardants and PCBs than their wild relatives.

In short: The quality of *our* food depends on the quality of the food we feed our animals and the way they are allowed to lead their lives.

It follows that, if we eat animal products, we need to make sure that the animals providing those foods are healthy and well-raised. We should reject *all* factory-farmed foods. We should reject meat or dairy from cattle fed other than grass and hay. We should reject the food industries' proposed solutions—such as radiation to kill bacteria—and instead we should make a commitment to only eat quality food. This is essential to our health and to quieting inflammation.

PRION DISEASES

There is yet another possible problem lurking in our food supply, that of prions. Prions are misshapen, infectious proteins. They act somewhat like viruses; they are highly contagious and are transmitted via body fluids. Prions are not heat sensitive and can neither be rendered away nor sterilized off surgical equipment. For example, variants of Creutzfeld Jacob's Disease (CJD), a human prion disease, have been transmitted during brain surgery and corneal transplantation, probably because prions contaminated surgical instruments despite sterilization. Children injected with human growth hormone developed and died from CJD.[3] Apparently, prions can be carried by hormones. Prions have their greatest impact on the brain where they cause tangles of nerves and vacuoles (holes) in the brain matter. Once infected, a person or animal loses their mind as well as their ability to eat, slowly wastes away and dies.

Prion diseases came to the public's attention in the 1990s when some Europeans developed mad cow disease after eating contaminated beef. Scientists immediately began searching for the cause of the upsurge in prion disease. They knew that a prion disease in sheep, scrapie, also causes holes and nerve tangles in sheep brains, giving rise to a fatal degenerative disease. Then scientists came across Kuru disease. The Kuru people ritually ate the brains of their dead relatives and subsequently developed the

---

[3] Only synthetic growth hormone is now used in children.

Kuru prion disease. This was the "aha moment," leading scientists to the conclusion that cannibalism plays a role in the development of prion diseases. At this point, many of us learned for the first time that cows were not fed grass and hay but instead were fed rendered cows. (Remember, high heat does not destroy prions.)

When mad cow disease first appeared in the United States, the federal government banned the feeding of cattle to cattle. However, the government only addressed ruminant feed; other animals are still fed their own species. Pigs are rendered and fed to pigs, chicken to chicken, turkey to turkey, farmed fish to farmed fish, mink to mink, and inadvertently pet to pet.[4] Pigs, chickens, sheep, fish, and turkeys fed cattle meat are fed back to cattle. Rendered feathers, hair, skin, hooves can also be found in feed, often under catch-all labels such as "animal protein products."

Any animal feed may incorporate swine, and poultry manure. This is troublesome in light of the recent discovery that cervids (deer, elk, and moose) excrete prions in their feces which may mean that feed made from manure may carry prions. There are also some who think that mad cow disease was caused by feeding cows sheep offal (the lower parts of sheep).

We are seeing new forms of prion diseases: We have mad cow disease (BSE, bovine spongiform encephalopathy) in cows and cattle; scrapie in sheep; CWD (chronic wasting disease) in deer, moose, and elk; FSE (feline spongiform encephalopathy) in cats; and TME (transmissible mink encephalopathy) in mink. Prions have been found in farmed fish. Pigs are also believed to have prion diseases. Nonetheless, we are told that prion diseases are on the decline and that we have nothing to worry about. However, some government actions indicate that troublesome issues remain:

Downer cows are cows that are not healthy enough to walk to slaughter. They have been eliminated from our food chain because they may be suffering from mad cow disease. A huge meat recall followed a Humane Society film showing cows being dragged to slaughter. This recall was not instigated because the government

---

[4]   Pet food manufacturers avoid "products" from smaller renderers who pick up dead animals from local veterinarians but the system is not perfect.

is concerned with the humane treatment of animals. In fact, the government permits other animals (sheep, pigs, etc.) to be dragged to slaughter. Instead, the meat was recalled because most of it was destined for the school lunch program. This suggests that a concern about the potential long-term effects of the meat.

The Japanese do not approve of how our cattle are raised. While our government does test for prions, less than two percent of the cattle entering the food chain are tested. Creekstone Farms, decided to prove that its cattle were prion-free by testing all of its cattle at its own expense. This plan ran aground when the USDA refused to sell them prion testing kits. The Federal Court of Appeals subsequently affirmed the USDA's right to prevent more widespread testing of meat.

In *Dying for a Hamburger*,[5] Murray Waldman, a Canadian coroner, makes an interesting statistical argument that early-onset Alzheimer's disease (a prion disease) is actually caused by prions from factory-farmed animals. Anyone who eats, or whose family eats, supermarket-quality animal products should read this book.

How to locate quality animal products

Quality animal products are available. They are increasingly easy to find at farmer's markets, in stores, and online. To ensure quality, we should only eat 100% grass-fed and grass-finished beef and dairy. We should only eat pasture-raised animal products, and our fish should be wild. Make sure (by asking questions) that the animals were not purchased from a feedlot, briefly pastured before slaughter, and then sold as grass-finished. Make sure animals were not merely fed grass for a period and then "finished" on grain and byproducts at a feedlot to be sold as grass- or range-fed. Do not be confused by labels that the meats are "natural" (this term has no meaning) or "vegetarian fed" (genetically modified corn is a vegetarian feed).

---

[5] Waldman M, Lamb M. *Dying for a Hamburger, Modern Meat Processing and the Epidemic of Alzheimer's Disease*. NY, NY: St. Martin's Press, 2005.

CHAPTER SUMMARY

The quality of what we eat is important. Look for properly raised meats, eggs, and dairy that are certified as humanely raised. Buy meats, eggs, and dairy products from reputable local farmers, buy shares in a Community Supported Agriculture (CSA) program, or buy your meats online directly from producers who explain in detail the quality of the products they sell. Remember, as Michael Pollan points out: We are not just what we eat, we are what what we eat eats as well.[6]

---

[6] Pollan M. *In Defense of Food.* N.Y., N.Y. Penguin Press 2008.

Chapter Eighteen
Glutathione

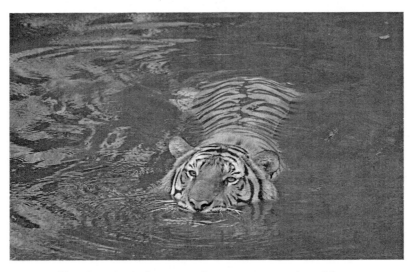

Simple, everyday exercise generates glutathione

Glutathione is a very simple molecule that contains sulfur groups that can bind mercury and other heavy metals. Glutathione is an end player in the oxidative stress game of hot potato. (See p. 97.) It helps "recycle" antioxidants that have donated electrons. Glutathione also helps our immune system fight infections more efficiently and prevent cancer. Glutathione levels are typically highest in healthy young people, lower in the healthy elderly, lower still in the ailing elderly, and lowest of all in the hospitalized elderly. Glutathione also enhances athletic performance. Athletes with adequate glutathione levels suffer less muscle damage, have better exercise recovery times, and show increased endurance.

Glutathione is made from three non-essential amino acids (cysteine, glycine, and glutamine). We can make non-essential amino acids from scratch so we do not have to get these three amino acids from diet (see chapter 16). However, we usually do not make them because they are widely present in our diet: Poultry, egg yolks, red peppers, garlic, onions, and Brussels sprouts provide cysteine. Fish, poultry, and beans contain glycine. Fish, eggs, cabbage, spinach, beans, parsley, and fermented foods provide glutamine. If we have adequate levels of B vitamins, we easily make glutathione. Foods rich in B vitamins include spinach, broccoli, lentils, turnip greens, and animal products.

We can also buy glutathione supplements. However, glutathione supplements are fairly expensive and the glutathione in them may be broken down into the three non-essential amino acids in the stomach. If that happens, the body must rebuild glutathione, in which case the supplement really is unnecessary.

CHAPTER SUMMARY

The best way to maintain healthy glutathione levels is simply to eat whole foods and exercise.

CHAPTER NINETEEN

Monosodium Glutamate (MSG)

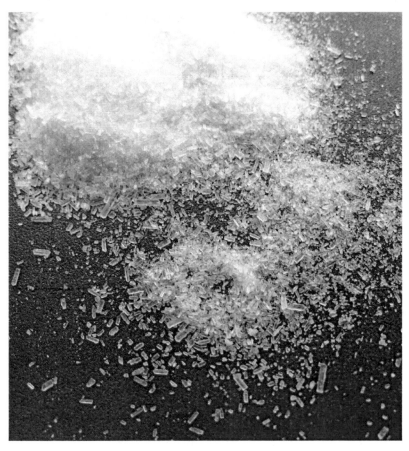

MSG Crystals

Monosodium glutamate (MSG) is the salt of an amino acid and is used as a food flavoring. We create small amounts of MSG in our bodies as we break down proteins. MSG also occurs naturally (again in small amounts) in many of the foods we eat. Larger amounts of MSG are also added to processed foods. There is a continuing debate about whether the additional MSG is bad for us or whether it is a safe, natural food flavoring.

Many individuals experience burning sensations along the back of the neck, chest tightness, nausea, sweating, and other symptoms that they attribute to eating foods with added MSG. These symptoms are often referred to as the "Chinese restaurant syndrome." Reactions to MSG vary. Some people report reactions to even very small amounts. MSG-induced reactions may occur immediately or up to 48 hours after the meal is eaten. There are reports that a subset of people with fibromyalgia improved dramatically when they excluded all forms of MSG from their food.

Ultimately, studies have failed to confirm that MSG causes adverse symptoms in any consistent manner. Instead, studies posit that the "Chinese restaurant syndrome" is an idiosyncratic reaction to shrimp, peanuts, spices, and other herbs in the food. The weight of the studies tends to show that MSG, at least in moderate amounts, is safe.[1]

There are, however, other studies that suggest that MSG may not be safe. Rats fed high amounts of MSG developed blindness and other visual problems. This study combined with epidemiological data showing an increased incidence of normal-tension glaucoma in certain parts of Asia (where a great deal of MSG is consumed) is troubling. Other studies link increased use

---

[1] Data on what constitutes a reasonable amount is lacking or very difficult to obtain.

of MSG with an increase in body mass (weight gain). The fact that MSG is used to develop obesity in rats (for research purposes) is also troubling. Finally, there is evidence that MSG does cause headaches and migraines, aggravates asthma, and causes other symptoms in some people.

We might elect to avoid MSG because its safety is not firmly established and because we gain no benefit from ingesting it. However, there are other important reasons why we should avoid MSG.

First, we are eating ever-increasing amounts of MSG but most of us are *not* consciously choosing to eat it. Almost all of the MSG we eat is "hidden" in our food.

Second, MSG is, as a rule, added to give poor-quality, nutritionally deficient food a more appealing taste. It is not added because it is good for us or because it makes good food better. It is used to trick our bodies, something we avoid as we work on quieting inflammation.

Hidden MSG

Much of the MSG we consume is "hidden" in our foods; technically speaking it is not added so it does not have to be listed as an ingredient on the label. Instead, we must learn which foods and chemicals come with MSG "built in" and *avoid them*.

MSG is always present in autolyzed yeast, calcium caseinate, gelatin, glutamate, glutamic acid, hydrolyzed corn gluten, hydrolyzed protein, monopotassium glutamate, monosodium glutamate, natrium glutamate, sodium caseinate, textured protein, yeast extract, yeast food, and yeast nutrient.

MSG is often present in anything protein fortified. It is usually found in barley malt, bouillon and broth, carrageenan, citric acid, flavors and flavorings, malt extract, malt flavoring, maltodextrin; natural beef, chicken, and pork flavoring; pectin, protease enzymes, seasonings, soy protein, soy protein concentrate, soy protein isolate, soy sauce, ultra-pasteurized dairy products, whey protein, whey protein concentrate, and whey protein isolate. Disodium guanylate and disodium inosinate are expensive food additives that work synergistically with inexpensive MSG. The presence of these two ingredients suggests that the product has MSG in it; they are rarely added to MSG-free foods.

In addition, there is the fairly new practice of renaming hydrolyzed proteins as pea protein, whey protein, corn protein, etc. If whole peas are a soup ingredient, the label must state that the soup contains peas. Calling an ingredient "pea protein" indicates that the pea has been hydrolyzed, at least in part, and that MSG is present. The fact that manufacturers feel the need to give hydrolyzed protein a more pleasant sounding name indicates that they are intentionally making it more difficult for people who read labels hoping to avoid non-foods or MSG.

Large amounts of MSG are often "hidden" in foods we eat. Note how many MSG-containing ingredients are in this veggie burger, one you might order at a fast food restaurant:[2]

VEGGIE BURGER INGREDIENTS:

Ingredients with MSG: Textured soy protein isolate * Calcium caseinate * Soy protein * Soy protein isolate * Autolyzed yeast extract * Natural flavors

Other ingredients: Egg white solids * Corn starch * Sugar * Wheat gluten * Salt, Spices, Garlic & Onion powder * Dextrose * Powdered peppers * Oils * Natural smoke flavor

---

This burger contains significant amounts of MSG to compensate for its lack of food ingredients. The MSG tricks your taste buds into thinking you are eating something substantial when, in fact, you are eating inexpensive chemicals. Likely when you ordered a non-meat patty and a salad, you did not plan to eat chemicals with MSG. This is why we must ask restaurants to provide ingredient lists for the foods they serve us. Most fast foods are high in MSG, chemicals, sugars, and genetically modified ingredients—which is yet another reason to avoid them. But many

---

[2] Many veggie burgers in your grocery store will contain similar ingredients, underscoring the importance of reading labels.

"better" restaurants also buy—and serve—processed foods in bulk that contain MSG, sugars, chemicals, etc.

MSG-carrying ingredients are also often added to many foods sold on popular weight-loss programs. In fact, before you sign on to a weight-loss plan, look carefully at the ingredients in the foods they offer to sell you. Ask yourself if the plan is concerned with your overall health. Are they suggesting you eat healthy foods or are they suggesting you lose weight by reducing calories and eating chemicals, including MSG, instead of whole foods? (See Appendix A, p. 275 for some examples of popular diet foods.)

CHAPTER SUMMARY

Opinions differ on whether MSG is bad for us. There is no question, however, but that MSG is used to make not-so-tasty ingredients taste better. There is also no question but that food manufacturers knowingly hide MSG in our food. With some frequency TV ads proclaim that certain soups or foods have no *added* MSG. The fine print moving across the TV screen then silently adds "except for the naturally occurring MSG in the autolyzed yeast, etc." Rather than unwittingly trick our taste buds into eating chemicals and poor quality food ingredients, we are going to avoid hidden MSG by eating only healthy, high quality, whole foods.

CHAPTER TWENTY

Genetically Modified Food

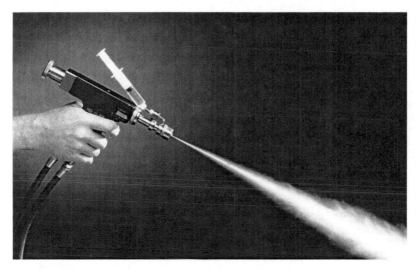

A gene gun used to modify animals

The safety of genetically modified (GM) food is far from settled. Many countries have decided that GM foods have not been proven safe. Others, such as Canada and the United States, are strongly in favor of the technique and see it as an important way to feed the world. While the debate continues, we need to understand, at the very least, what is involved and the potential negative consequences of eating GM foods.

Genetic modification is often presented as a "gene splicing" technique. This conjures up the image of a precise technique where scientists are able to enter a cell (invisible to the naked eye), enter the yet smaller nucleus, and cut open the DNA of that cell to insert a gene in a specific spot. Our technology cannot do this.

Most plants are instead modified using a "gene gun" to blast genes into the plant's DNA. Thousands of tiny shards (nano particles) of gold or tungsten are coated with the foreign genes. These coated shards are placed on the barrel of the gene gun that shoots them at a petri dish containing thousands of plant cells.

Some of the genes will—by chance—end up in the right place on some of the DNA. Some genes will end up on the "wrong" place on the DNA, damaging genes in ways that cannot be identified (or ruled out) at present. Most of the genes will end up in the cell's cytoplasm (the larger part of the cell surrounding the nucleus). In order to modify the plant, the gene must be in the plant's DNA in a way that can be expressed and passed on to future generations. Of course, it is impossible to tell by looking which of the many plant cells in the petri dish have been successfully modified.

This dilemma was resolved by adding another gene to the first. An antibiotic-resistant marker (ARM) is attached to the first gene, and both genes are then shot at the plant cells. Next, the petri dish is doused with a toxic amount of antibiotic. Any cells that survive are expressing the gene for antibiotic resistance. This means they also have the "target" gene (usually for herbicide resistance) in their DNA. It also means that GM foods usually contain a gene for antibiotic resistance. For instance, GM corn modified to produce an insecticidal compound (Bt or *Bacillus thuringiensis)* also has a gene for resistance to the antibiotic ampicillin.

Many scientists worry that, when humans and animals eat GM food, antibiotic-resistant marker genes will transfer to the intestinal flora, creating new strains of antibiotic-resistant bacteria. The British Medical Association mentioned this risk as a reason for requesting an immediate moratorium on genetically engineered foods. In response, the biotech industry cited animal studies showing that DNA does not survive digestion. However, subsequent studies found DNA in the blood, liver, spleen, and feces of test animals. In another study, volunteers ate a fast-food hamburger and milkshake that contained GM soy. The herbicide-resistant gene in the soy was transferred to intestinal bacteria after a single meal. Given that *all* fast food contains GM products, and given that tens of millions of people eat tens of millions of fast food meals daily, the ARM technique used to produce GM foods may well be adding to the very real problems of antibiotic resistance that we are struggling with at present.

Unpredictability

"Genetic engineering is generally a hit-and-miss affair. The genes may be inserted the wrong way round or multiple copies may be scattered throughout a plant's genome. They may be inserted inside other genes—destroying their activity or massively increasing it. More worryingly, a plant's genetic make-up may become unstable—again with unpredictable results ... Rogue toxins may be produced or existing ones amplified massively. Such problems may only arise hundreds of generations after the crops are originally modified." [1]

Another concern with genetic modification is our inability to predict how these new genes will express themselves in the future.

---

[1] Smith Jeffrey M. *Genetic Roulette: The Documented Health Risks of Genetically Engineered Foods.* White River Jct., VT: Chelsea Green Publishing, 2007.

In Scotland, work was underway to genetically modify salmon to create a fish that grew more quickly. This work derailed for a while when the new gene began to turn the salmon meat green—an unintended (and undesirable) side effect of the new gene.[2]

In another experiment, a gene was added to make petunias a deeper red. However, when the modified seeds were planted in a field, the flowers that grew were not all red. They varied in both color and pattern. They also changed depending on various environmental factors (season, etc.), showing that the effect of the new gene was unpredictable.

A different technique is used to modify bacteria which then produce drugs and other chemicals, a technique that is approved in most countries. This method was used by a manufacturer of tryptophan, an amino acid used as a supplement to promote sleep. The GM bacteria produced tryptophan, and the tryptophan was encapsulated and marketed. Subsequently, reports of deaths and permanent nerve damage began surfacing among those taking this tryptophan supplement. The bacteria produced tryptophan as planned but also, for unknown reasons, produced a neurotoxin.[3]

A POTENTIAL PROBLEM WITH GM CANOLA

The examples above show that we cannot with certainty guarantee what genes a modified plant or animal may express or how they may express them. This uncertainty poses particular problems in plants that already have genes for toxins. Take canola for instance: The rape plant carries a gene that produces erucic acid. Erucic acid is a toxin that can cause fatty degeneration of the heart and adrenals. The rape plant was hybridized and a strain was created that produces very little erucic acid—but the gene for the toxin remains in the rape plants. Now, some 50 percent of the rape plants are grown from genetically modified seed. Will these plants at some point begin producing much greater amounts of erucic acid? We do not know. When we consume conventional canola

---

[2] Subsequently, salmon was successfully modified and is expected to be approved in the near future.

[3] In response, governments banned the sale of tryptophan; they did not withdraw their approval of the modification technique used.

oil, we are relying on spot checks of the crops to ensure that the oil does not contain excessive amounts of erucic acid. We must decide if we wish to rely on those safeguards or not.

POTENTIAL ISSUES WITH SYNTHETIC BOVINE GROWTH HORMONE (BGH)

The first genetically modified food to enter our food chain was dairy from cows injected with synthetic bovine growth hormone (BGH). BGH was developed to increase milk production and is injected in cows twice a month.

After injection, the growth hormone levels in the cow's blood may jump to around 1,000 times normal levels. After reviewing this data, the FDA proposed regulations that milk could not be sold for five days after a BGH injection and meat from the cow could not be sold for ten days after injection.[4] Having to dump close to one-third (ten days' worth) of the milk produced in a month, of course, would prevent the injection from increasing milk production. The dairy industry convinced the FDA to abandon the proposed regulation based on a showing that humans do not absorb cow growth hormone.

This did not, however, satisfy the safety concerns of some (such as European oversight agencies) because an increase in growth hormone also increases the production of IGF-1 (insulin-like growth factor 1). Cow and human IGF-1 are very similar. It is not destroyed by pasteurization, and humans can absorb cow IGF-1. IGF-1 is a very strong hormone and causes cells to divide. Elevated level of IGF-1 in humans has been linked to both breast and prostate cancers as well as colon, lung, and others. We do not need extra IGF-1.

We do not know if the jump in growth hormone and IGF-1 in cows is due to the concentrated amounts of hormone used in the twice-monthly injections or is due to the genetic modification of the hormone. In Europe, many countries opted to avoid BGH until these questions were answered and the hormone was proven safe. Other countries, the United States among them, opted to assume the hormone was safe.

---

[4] Growth hormone has an affinity for muscle, hence the proposed longer delay for the sale of muscle (or meat) from cows slaughtered shortly after BGH injection.

BGH poses other problems in animals. Rats fed BGH developed an antibody response to the hormone. Cows injected with BGH suffer from birth defects, reproductive disorders, increased incidence of mastitis, foot and leg injuries, indigestion, bloat, diarrhea, and shortened lives. The pus content of milk from BGH cows was shown to increase another 19 percent compared with the milk of untreated cows. These are independent reasons to consider avoiding BGH dairy products.

OTHER GENETICALLY MODIFIED FOODS

Most vegetable oils used in restaurant and processed foods are made from soy, corn, canola, or cottonseed oil. Substantial portions of these crops are grown from genetically modified seed. The potential problems with GM canola are discussed above.

Sixty percent of our exposure to GM products comes from corn and soy. At least 80% of the soy, 40% of corn, 60% of canola, and 70% of cottonseed grown in the United States are GM. These crops are often present in processed foods. Fifty percent of Hawaiian papaya is GM while papaya from other regions is not. In 2009, GM sugar entered our food chain.[5] Today, several new countries are working on developing other GM foods. One of the most active in this arena is China, where work is being done on modified wheat and rice, among other crops. Europe and other countries have disapproved GM foods because they consider the safety data supporting approval in North America to be insufficient and unreliable. Many of us have serious concerns about China's safety record. In one instance, people were sickened because the pesticide residue on some foods grown in China was approximately 37,000 times over the legal limit. Then there was the melamine contamination of powdered milk that sickened infants and melamine contamination of pet food that killed numerous cats and dogs. Can we rely on Chinese data showing that their new GM foods are safe? This is of great concern because

---

[5] In 2010, a federal district court judge temporarily halted further planting of GM sugar beets but sugar from beets planted before that ruling went into effect are not affected by the ruling.

China now produces significant amounts of the foods we eat and is busily working on creating new GM crops.

AVOIDING GM FOODS

You likely have noticed that the produce in grocery stores today all carry little stickers with numbers on them. These PLU (price look-up) numbers are used to identify the type of produce (a gala apple [4133], a Granny Smith apple [4107], a small lemon [4033], etc.). They also identify how the produce was grown. Produce that is grown conventionally, such as those above, carry stickers with four numbers. Produce with a sticker carrying five numbers, always beginning with a "9," is certified organic. An apple with a sticker reading 94133 is an organic gala apple. The original PLU number system also included an "8" that would have

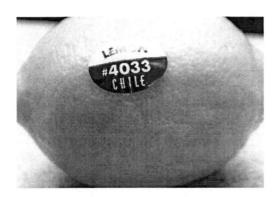

told us that the produce was genetically modified. The "8" system has been abandoned, and there is no easy way to tell if conventional produce is GM or not. This, of course, makes it more difficult to avoid GM produce. Fortunately, most produce presently is not GM. However, this may change rapidly.

CHAPTER SUMMARY

In other countries, any food that contains a GM ingredient must state that fact on the food's label. In North America, the manufacturer may choose not to inform consumers that their product is made from GM ingredients—and they consistently choose not to include this information on their labels. If you decide you wish to avoid GM foods, you must:

1. Learn which foods in the market may be genetically modified. There are websites, such as http://www.ucsusa.org/food_and_ agriculture/science_and_impacts/science/engineered-foods-allowed-on.html where you can try to gain this information.[6] Only buy those foods if they are certified organic (which prohibits the use of any genetically modified ingredients—including the feeding of GM corn to cows—in organic food).

2. Buy locally, where you can speak to the producer/grower and verify that no GM inputs are used.

3. Contact the manufacturer of a product you are interested in purchasing to ensure they are not using GM inputs. If they do not respond, assume they are using GM inputs.

> To understand the prevalence of GM foods, consider the following information from a United States government site: "In 2006, 252 million acres of [GM] crops were planted in 22 countries by 10.3 million farmers. The majority of these crops were herbicide- and insect-resistant soybeans, corn, cotton, canola, and alfalfa. Other crops grown commercially or field-tested are a sweet potato resistant to a virus ... rice with increased iron and vitamins ... and a variety of plants able to survive weather extremes ...
>
> On the horizon are bananas that produce human vaccines against infectious diseases such as hepatitis B; fish that mature more quickly; cows that are resistant to bovine spongiform encephalopathy (mad cow disease); fruit and nut trees that yield years earlier, and plants that produce new plastics with unique properties."
>
> http://www.ornl.gov/sci/techresources/ Human_Genome/elsi/gmfood.shtml March 2010.

---

[6] It is actually very difficult to track down this information. The FDA does not presently publish lists of approved GM crops.

Chapter Twenty-One
Frequently Asked Questions

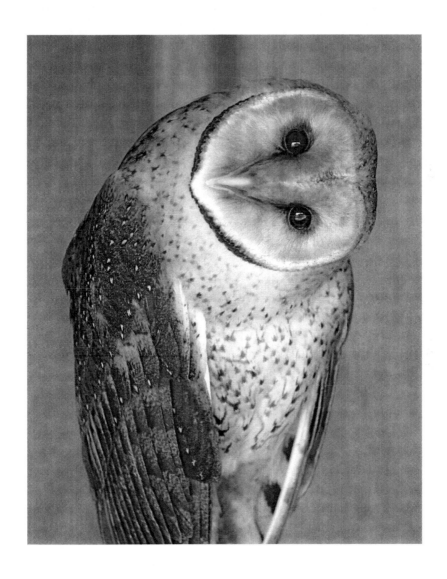

Yes. This plan eliminates chemicals, bad fats, sweeteners and added sugars, genetically modified ingredients, and cuts back on high omega-6 foods. It also helps us avoid xenoestrogens, persistent toxins, and heavy metals. Children are more sensitive to those things than adults are, and benefit more when they are eliminated from the diet.

The plan adds significant amounts of whole fruits and vegetables filled with vitamins, antioxidants, phytoestrogens, phytosterols (plant fats), and other beneficial compounds that children need. The whole foods on the plan are healthy and children need them.

The plan limits the proportionate amount of protein in the diet but easily provides enough protein for a child to thrive without providing an excess that will burden the child's liver, kidneys, and bones. Many websites provide detailed information on the protein needs of growing children; one is http://www.cdc.gov/nutrition/everyone/basics/protein.html. Take a look at one if you are concerned about how much protein your children are eating. The plan limits dairy but studies show that children do not need dairy as a protein or calcium source as long as they eat an otherwise healthy diet. Of course, a dairy-sensitive child will do much better without dairy.

Adults may not graze or eat bedtime snacks on the plan. Because growing children have bursts of growth hormone throughout the day, children and growing teenagers are allowed healthy snacks, including bedtime snacks, as desired.

The trick with children, since they are often rigid about what they will and will not eat, is to make sure that they are getting enough calories and good fats in their diet as well as enough variety of fruits and vegetables. Often, if the child has already developed poor eating habits—and has acquired a taste for fast foods and sugar —changes will have to be made gradually. However, a parent aware of the amount of persistent toxins in animal products, and aware of the greater effect xenoestrogens have on a child, can become quite persuasive about the need to change.

Teenagers are typically most difficult. With them, parents

are limited to controlling what is served in the home and often have to wait for peer pressure to recede, and the teen's sense of invincibility to pass, before the teenager will change. This often does not happen until the child is well into adulthood.

Healthy diets for children would be vastly improved if we could improve school lunches. One big obstacle is that the federal government subsidizes the food industry through large purchases of surplus foods for the school lunch program. Thus, most beef recalls have been of poor-quality meat destined for the school lunches. When swine flu decreased the demand for pork products, the government stepped in and significantly increased pork purchases, again for the school lunch program. Concern that foods be free of toxins, chemicals, and sugars is generally lacking. Certainly this is an arena where parents should become much more proactive. We should also work on changing college food programs where young adults are required to pre-purchase truly poor-quality food and often cannot make any substitutions

Is this plan healthy for pregnant or nursing women?

Yes, as long as their health care providers approve their dietary changes, and two other issues are addressed. Pregnant and lactating women have very different hormones circulating than the average adult does. They also have increased calorie needs. They should eat as their appetite dictates, including additional snacks during the day and at bedtime, if desired. They also must make sure that they eat enough to satisfy their need for additional calories.

In all other respects, the plan is healthy because it helps them avoid chemicals and toxins that may be detrimental to the growing fetus or nursing child. It also ensures that their food is rich in all of the nutrients needed for healthy growth and development.

What is too much exercise in terms of oxidative stress?

There is really no such thing as "too much exercise." When we exercise, we transform stored energy into a usable energy and that conversion generates free radicals. If you exercise vigorously more than an hour a day, you need to add extra antioxidants to your diet to help quiet the free radicals generated. Of course, as you exercise you also generate detoxifying compounds but you will still need to increase both your caloric as well as your nutrient intake at or about the time you exercise. In other words, a vigorous

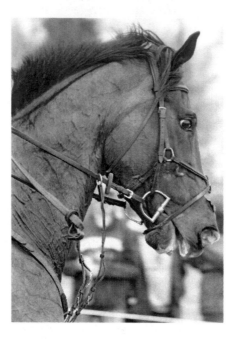

Exercise can generate free radicals

work out should be followed by a very healthy meal or snack. You can also help offset the extra free radicals generated by exercise by being more careful about avoiding refined foods, bad fats, and chemicals.

I EXERCISE A LOT. HOW SHOULD I EAT TO AVOID REDUCED PERFORMANCE?

If you exercise more than an hour a day, you should do the following to avoid fatigue:

1. Eat something before exercise (like fruits and nuts). Provide your body with nutrients but not so much that you create digestive issues that will interfere with your workout.

2. During an endurance event/training, you may need to replace your sugar stores and electrolytes as you go. Continue to use aids that you have used in the past during events (sugar gels, electrolytes, etc.) but look for products without strange colorings and chemicals.

3. Immediately after a workout, your body is primed to replenish your glycogen stores—critical to your next workout. You need carbohydrates and protein in a ratio of about 4:1 or so and this should be eaten within a half hour of your work out. This meal is more important than stretching. Think high-glycemic vegetables (baked sweet potatoes, carrots), think blueberries, some nuts, humus. You do not need refined carbs to maintain your strength, in fact, your body also needs the antioxidants and other nutrients provided by these foods.

4. You must maintain your calorie intake over a day because your workouts burn calories. This means that coconut milk, nuts, seeds, nut butters, avocados, well-made mayos, pesto made without cheese, guacamole, and such need to be a big part of your diet. You need to toss both your vegetables and your fish (or whatever protein you choose) in sauces and dips. Again, you can provide your body with both the calories and the nutrients you need without switching to the refined carbs and sugars many athletes rely on.

5. You may freely eat fruit but neither fruit nor vegetables alone will provide you enough calories to sustain demanding workouts.

Serious body builders should eat this way as well. Such workouts may somewhat increase your need for protein but surprisingly, your protein needs do not jump dramatically (see http://indoorclimbing.com).

WHAT CAUSES LEG CRAMPS?

There are many potential causes of leg cramps and it may take some experimenting to overcome them. Common causes include:

1. Lack or imbalance of calcium.
2. Lack or imbalance of magnesium.
3. Dehydration.
4. Lack or imbalance of sodium or other electrolytes.
5. Overhydration.

Dark leafy greens, nuts, and other plant foods are fabulous sources of calcium, magnesium, and other electrolytes. If you are used to eating a lot of dairy and are not yet eating many leafy greens, you may need additional calcium, perhaps as a supplement.

Most Americans are deficient in magnesium, so you may need more magnesium. See chapter 12 for information on foods rich in magnesium. Sometimes magnesium supplements are useful.

Many people avoid water and herbal teas before bed to avoid waking during the night to go to the bathroom. This can lead to dehydration. You may simply need to increase your fluid intake in the hours before going to bed to avoid nightly muscle cramps. Caffeinated and alcoholic beverages can increase dehydration and thus may aggravate the situation.

Athletes who sweat profusely lose sodium from their bodies. Many no longer eat processed foods and do not salt their food. Leg cramps may occur if there is a sodium deficiency.

Some people force themselves to drink large amounts of water. Water in excess can dilute the mineral levels in our blood and lead to cramping. If you are eating a lot of fresh fruit and vegetables, you may find that reducing your water intake somewhat (not so much as to cause dehydration), may help alleviate your leg cramps. Over-hydration occurs more in athletes who drink water to replace fluid lost as sweat, but who do not replenish potassium and sodium also lost.

If your leg cramps persist and are very severe, you should check with your health care provider as various illnesses, as well as certain prescription drugs, can cause leg cramps.

MY STOOLS ARE VERY LOOSE, WHAT SHOULD I DO?

First, make sure you are replacing lost fluid to prevent dehydration.

Diarrhea is often treated by eliminating wheat, dairy, and greasy foods, something we are already doing. In terms of what may be causing the problem: Sometimes the shift to a high-fiber diet overwhelms the intestinal tract unused to the fiber and populated with microbes not so capable of processing fiber. Shifting back to a diet lower in fiber and then gradually increasing fiber can be helpful. Some people find that removing the skins, seeds, and membranes from fruits and vegetables makes these foods easier to digest. Canned or well-cooked fruits and vegetables may also be easier to digest.

Eliminating foods such as legumes (e.g., lentils, kidney beans, lima beans), peas, corn, broccoli, spinach, and eating fewer nuts for a while may help. If gas or cramping is an issue, it can be helpful to avoid dried peas and beans, broccoli, cabbage, cauliflower, onions, and Brussels sprouts.

It also helps to evaluate the amount of fructose in the diet. Often, people radically increase their consumption of fruit and sweet vegetables during the first weeks on the plan. Excess fructose is fermented in the colon and can cause a great deal of intestinal distress, so consider eating fewer apples, apricots, cantaloupes and other melons, grapes, peaches, and pears. Instead, choose kiwi, berries, bananas, and citrus.

Also look at the amount of raw vegetables or fruit you are eating as they, initially, can be a source of the problem. This is especially true if there is underlying intestinal inflammation. Raw vegetables and fruit contain more rough cellular tissue, and the inflamed intestinal mucous membrane may not be ready for roughage. Even one small fresh cucumber may lead to very unpleasant consequences the next morning. Be cautious with raw vegetables and fruit after diarrhea. Spicy dishes may also aggravate.

Finally, consider whether you have increased the amount of a food that you may be sensitive to: Common culprits include soy, shellfish, and tree nuts.

For most, increasing fluid intake and reducing the amount of fruit and raw vegetables will provide significant relief. Sometimes taking psyllium seed as a supplement can speed up this process. Of course, you need to make sure that you do not have an underlying infection and that you are drinking enough fluids.

I AM CONSTIPATED, WHAT SHOULD I DO?

Usually, increasing the amount of fiber in the diet works to cure constipation. If the opposite is true for you, the first step is to make sure you are drinking enough water and other fluids. Try warm liquids, especially in the morning.

Sometimes, eliminating dairy can cause constipation in a person who is sensitive to dairy. There, the inflammatory effect of dairy has caused stools to soften, resulting in a rebound problem when dairy is eliminated. Sometimes, when dairy is removed, people drink less coffee in the morning and the usual trigger for a bowel movement is missing. Try nut milks in your coffee instead of eliminating it.

Psyllium as a supplement, if combined with enough fluids, can also help in constipation. The psyllium seeds will pull water into the colon, softening the stool. Also, consider whether you are eating more of a food that you may be sensitive to that is triggering a constipative response. Occasionally, constipation can be caused by too much fructose in the fruit we eat.

You should contact your health care provider if this is a new problem for you, if you have blood in your stool, if you have severe pain with bowel movements, or if your constipation lasts more than two weeks.

HOW DO I KNOW IF I AM GETTING ALL THE NUTRIENTS I NEED?

There are numerous websites that help you calculate the amount of protein and other nutrients you are getting from your diet. One of the best ways to learn the nutrient content of a particular food is to use the U.S. government's website: http://www.nal.usda.gov/fnic/foodcomp/search. This database seems a bit complex at first but provides reliable, neutral, and detailed information. Using it, you first search for a particular food. Then you put in the quantity of the food you are eating. Although the website suggests an amount (for instance, a cup or a medium-sized piece of fruit), you can change the amount so you can get information for the exact amount of the food you are eating.

SHOULD I CONTINUE TAKING SUPPLEMENTS?

This plan is about using food to quiet inflammation. Whether we also should take supplements, and if so which ones, is beyond the scope of the plan. I recommend that you continue taking what you have been taking and that you ask for advice on taking additional supplements from a trained health care professional familiar with your individual needs. That said, a multi-vitamin certainly might be useful to ensure that you are getting needed nutrients as you work on changing your eating habits.

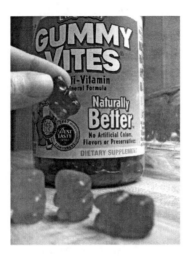

I do have two general comments: Your supplements should not contain added sugar, chemicals, and strange fillers, additives, and colors. If yours do, look for a better-quality supplement. And remember, you often get what you pay for and the cheapest supplement available may not be the best supplement.

There is often a difference between bio-identical supplements and chemically produced versions. All biological compounds have a rotation that is necessary for function. In nature, they always rotate to the right. Bio-identical supplements also rotate to the right. When compounds are made in a laboratory, half of what is made will rotate to the right and the other half will rotate left. That other half, designated by "l" (for levro, Latin for left) on the label, cannot be used by the body and may even be damaging. Thus, a bottle of vitamin E that contains dl-alpha tocopherol contains a synthetic version of one of the compounds that makes up the E complex our body needs. A bottle of mixed tocopherols and tocotrienes, all with the designation "d" (for dextro, Latin for right), is a more complete, natural form of vitamin E that will work better than the laboratory created dl-alpha tocopherol.

Finally, it is wise to learn all you can about how vitamins actually are produced. The book *Twinkie Deconstructed*[1] explains

---

[1] Ettlinger S. *Twinkie, Deconstructed*. NY, NY: Hudson Street Press, 2007.

that some vitamins are produced in China using petrochemicals as a start. I highly recommend reading this book, as the knowledge you gain about how our food chemicals and vitamins are made may motivate you to work harder on getting the nutrients you need from whole foods.

MAY I TAKE MY SUPPLEMENTS BEFORE BED?

In the wild, we would get our vitamins from our food. Because other compounds in our food may help us use and absorb vitamins, it seems logical to take vitamins with meals rather than before bed. In addition, many supplements contain small amounts of sugars, fats, and gelatin so it is preferable not to take them in the fasting period two to three hours before bed.

However, if you have a prescription or supplement that is to be taken before bed, you need to follow those recommendations. This is also true if your health care provider wants you to eat something when you take a prescription at bedtime. Follow that advice, but do make sure that your choice of food is low-glycemic and low-insulinemic in order to minimize the negative effect on your nocturnal burst of growth hormone (see p. 47).

CAN I TEST MY LEVELS OF INFLAMMATORY CYTOKINES?

It is possible to measure the blood levels of various cytokines. However, the information on cytokine levels is not yet well-standardized in terms of laboratory techniques and value ranges. Nor, because of the complexity of the immune system, is there a good understanding of what an out-of-range value for any particular cytokine means. Physicians typically do not order cytokine tests and insurance companies do not usually reimburse for these tests because the results do not have sufficient diagnostic value. At present, the best standard marker for inflammation in the body is reflected by the C-reactive protein test. This marker, when high, indicates that a person is inflamed but does not identify the cause. Homocysteine levels are used similarly.

There are laboratories online that will test for inflammatory cytokines such as Interleukin-6 (Il-6) or tumor necrosis factor a (TNF-a). But again, the meaning of the results from those tests remains unclear. For instance, if unbeknownst to you, you are fighting off a virus, your cytokine levels might be high causing you to assume incorrectly that you are overly inflamed. Or those you test for may be in the normal range while others not tested are not.

Do you recommend milk thistle supplements?

No, milk thistle is not a supplement that everyone needs. Milk thistle capsules contain a concentrated amount of an antioxidant complex found only in small amounts in milk thistle seed. These compounds show many interesting benefits: For instance, they help protect the liver and kidneys from damage and they may protect the skin from oxidative stress damage. But as these are isolated, concentrated plant compounds, only a person trained in the use of botanicals will know if these supplements are appropriate for you.

In contrast, whole milk thistle seed, which you can buy in bulk at health food stores, can from time to time be used as a tea or ground, sprinkled on food (although some find it too tough raw even when ground), or baked into muffins. Russian studies indicate that milk thistle seed used this way helps protect the liver in a gentle way. We might all benefit from including "wild foods," such as milk thistle seed, in our diet from time to time.

Does glucosamine have sugar in it?

Glucosamine is derived from glucose but the two chemicals follow different metabolic pathways in the body. Taking glucosamine does not directly affect blood sugar levels but you should still inform your health care provider that you are taking this supplement if you are diabetic.

Interestingly, there is some evidence based on both human and animal studies that glucosamine may increase insulin resistance if taken over a long period. Ideally, eating to quiet inflammation will relieve the need for the use of glucosamine for the long term.

QUESTIONS ABOUT FOOD

MAY I EAT RED MEAT WHILE I AM TESTING FOR FOOD SENSITIVITIES?

No, if you are testing foods, you should be on the Elimination Phase. This phase limits the intake of cholesterol and persistent toxins. Its ability to quiet inflammation will be altered if you are eating additional animal products.

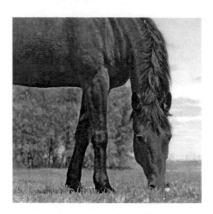

Avoid grazing

I TEND TO STRETCH OUT MY MEALS. IS THAT OKAY?

From time-to-time it is fine to have a leisurely meal where you linger over the food and enjoy good company. Most meals, however, should have a beginning and an end that are not too far apart. Otherwise, you are simply grazing. A meal should not be stretched out by doing work in between bites. If you tend to do that, set a limit on how long a meal is (15 minutes for a snack, 30 minutes for lunch, 45 minutes, at most, for dinner). When that time has passed, quit eating even if you are not done, even if you are still hungry. When the next meal or snack rolls around, you will likely be hungry enough to finish it more quickly.

MUST I EAT TWO DAILY SNACKS?

Yes, during the Elimination Phase you must eat two snacks a day. They can be as small as you like, but they must be eaten. Many of us have a pattern of not eating simply because we often are too busy and do not want to take the time to eat. This means that we are not eating even though our bodies would prefer that we did. Eating snacks is a way of forcing us to listen to our bodies.

After the Elimination and Testing Phases you may begin to eliminate snacks if you are normal weight. If you are underweight, you should continue eating snacks. Be careful if you are overweight, as often the liver is unable to properly maintain blood sugar levels. Not eating regularly can result in overwhelming food cravings that make it very difficult to eat healthfully.

Is salt intake limited on the plan?

The typical Western diet is high in processed foods and very high in salt. Once you start eating real foods, your salt intake usually plummets even if you salt your food at the table. This plan does not limit salt intake because most people who do not eat processed foods easily ingest less than a teaspoon of salt a day, the ideal upper limit for salt intake, even if they use salt for flavor.

One concern with salt is that it will tend to raise blood pressure. In fact, few people are salt sensitive, meaning that reasonable amounts of salt will not raise their blood pressure. Of course, there are exceptions to every rule. If you have high blood pressure and have been advised to avoid salt, by all means continue to do so. There are many good veggie salts on the market that you can use to season your food. If you simply want to make sure salt does not adversely affect your blood pressure, you should take your blood pressure frequently, and observe whether your blood pressure rises when you salt your food. If it does, cut back on your salt intake. If it does not, do not worry about the salt in your whole foods diet but do worry about the salt in any processed, packaged foods you continue to eat or if you eat out frequently. In those cases, the salt content is usually high, the offsetting plant nutrients and fluids are usually lacking, and salt becomes a health issue.

If you exercise a great deal—and sweat—you need to replenish the electrolytes you lose in your sweat, including sodium. You may need to add some salt to your food to avoid muscle cramping.

Are foods better raw or cooked?

Many advocates of raw foods argue that a raw food is healthier because cooking denatures enzymes needed to properly digest food. I am not deeply impressed with this argument.

Enzymes are proteins, and cooking denatures proteins. When we grind up food with our molars, we release proteolytic enzymes that help break down the food we are eating. As we chew our food, we release our own salivary enzymes that also help break down the plant material we are eating. When we swallow, our food is plunged into an acid bath in our stomach that denatures many of the plant enzymes in the food we swallowed. The journey from the mouth to the stomach is short, and the body's use of food-contained enzymes for digestion is generally rather short-lived.

Exceptions exist. For instance, the plant enzyme myrosinase converts compounds in the cabbage family to more potent, beneficial compounds and appears not to be denatured by stomach acid. While intestinal bacteria also provide myrosinase, cooking may diminish our absorption of certain beneficial compounds in the cabbage family. I would place a strong emphasis on the word "may" in the preceding sentence. It is highly unlikely that we need to rely on enzymes in our food for proper digestion; instead we can manage well using our own enzymes and those of our intestinal flora.[2] Moreover, as we cut up our food before cooking, plant enzymes are released and go to work, so we may gain the benefit they provide by simply letting cut vegetables sit for a little while before cooking them.

It is, however, true that antioxidants and other important compounds are affected by how we process our food. The fresher the food, the more nutrients it will contain. As our food sits around or is shipped long distances, it loses nutrients. On the other hand, food grown locally in nutrient-poor soil may contain fewer nutrients than food shipped from afar. Freezing preserves many nutrients by slowing down the aging process. As a result, frozen foods may be more nutrient-dense than a droopy fresh specimen, even if locally grown.

When we cook foods, we do destroy some compounds: Vitamin C diminishes as we heat our food. On the other hand, cooking tomatoes makes their lycopene more easily absorbed. Solanine, a

---

2   Some people do not make enough digestive enzymes. These people often benefit more from digestive aids, like bitters, than from a raw food diet.

troublesome alkaloid in nightshades (tomatoes, potatoes, eggplant, and peppers) is reduced and agaratine, a carcinogenic compound found in some mushrooms is destroyed by heat, reducing the potential toxicity of some foods.

Some foods, such as meats and fish, are prone to bacterial contamination, spoilage, and worms that are killed by heat. On the other hand, cooking animal products tends to generate carcinogens such as heterocyclic amines and benzo[a]pyrenes. Whether a particular food is better raw or cooked may depend entirely on which of the thousands of compounds in that food are under consideration. It also appears to vary greatly from study to study. There are studies showing that raw cabbage is far superior to steamed cabbage. Others show them to be equivalent. All of those studies show boiled cabbage to be near worthless, yet other studies show boiled cabbage to be filled with valuable nutrition.

For most of us, the big issue is not whether our food should be raw or cooked. Instead, our big challenge is to eat nutritious foods in the right proportions. A raw foods diet can be a very healthy choice, but only in a person who works diligently to create a varied diet that does not include smoothies and concoctions that are drunk rather than chewed. For most people, a cooked diet rich in whole foods will be the most practical, healthy choice.

Since there are pros and cons to any preparation method, we may do well to be informed by our own preferences. Which tastes better to you: Cooked or raw carrots, onions, tomatoes? Your innate preferences may indicate individual nutrient needs or individual inabilities to process certain compounds in a food prepared a certain way.

SHOULD I EAT RAW MUSHROOMS?

Most of the mushrooms we eat, the little white or brown ones and the larger portabello mushrooms, belong to the Agaricus family. Members of this family have a tendency to produce a carcinogenic compound called agaratine. Agaratine breaks down in cooking, so mycologists (mushroom specialists) recommend cooking mushrooms. Also, mushrooms are odd and we do not know as much as we should about all of the compounds in them.

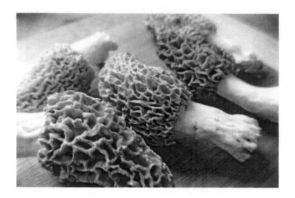

To avoid potential problems, mycologists recommend that we not eat any raw mushrooms, even if they are not in the Agaricus family. As they are expert, I follow their advice but I have in the past eaten raw mushrooms and survived. I do, however, think that cooked mushrooms have a superior taste.

SHOULD NUTS BE RAW?

Your nuts may be raw, roasted, and/or salted as long as they are not roasted in prohibited or poor-quality oils.

WHY ARE FRESH AND DRIED VEGETABLES OFTEN TREATED DIFFERENTLY?

Fresh corn counts as a vegetable. Dried corn counts as a grain and is not allowed during the Elimination Phase. Fresh green beans, including edamame and green limas, count as a vegetable. Dried soy, lima, and other dried legumes count as protein.

Often different varieties of corn and beans are used for growing fresh and dried vegetables. Their characteristics and their uses are different. As a result, they are treated differently.

QUESTIONS ABOUT FATS

ARE FATS LIMITED ON THE PLAN?

This plan does not limit the amount of good fats in the diet. Instead, it eliminates all poor-quality fats. Good fats are important and we seldom overeat them. We control the overall fat content of the diet by making olive oil our primary oil, as few of us drink olive oil by the cup. Other fats and oils are used as taste enhancers, which means we do not make desserts using cups of coconut milk, instead we use coconut milk to add flavor and mouth feel to our fruits and vegetables. We do not always use coconut oil for sautéing; we use it occasionally for flavor. Even if we eat dairy, we do not fry our food in butter nor do we make sauces out of it; instead we might occasionally put a pat of butter on a baked potato. As long as we follow these rules, and most of our fat is in the form of olive oil, there is no need to worry about fats in the diet.

How do I know if an oil is deodorized or solvent extracted?

Generally speaking, we need to spend some time finding out how the oils we use are processed. Manufacturers whose oils are carefully processed typically make a point of explaining the care they take to make a superior oil. They are more than happy to explain or answer questions about their products. Most manufacturers have websites where you can ask questions and get product information. Take advantage of those options. Health food stores, such as Whole Foods and local cooperatives, also have sites that cover these topics. A little research reveals that most grapeseed and rice bran oils are hexane extracted. Hexane is a toxic solvent that you should avoid. Similarly, avocado oil is often solvent extracted. The health food store sites will help you find brands of these oils that are neither refined nor extracted with solvents.

Are the saturated fats in coconut oil a problem?

This plan allows the use of coconut oil. While olive oil is our main oil, coconut oil may be used as an occasional high-heat cooking oil or to add flavor to vegetable dishes.

Coconut oil is a saturated plant oil. Some health care practitioners recommend avoiding saturated fats. As so often is the case, the jury is still out on whether all types of saturated fats (or any saturated fats) affect us adversely. Butter and other animal products contain saturated fats built from palmitic and myristic acids, types of saturated fats that have been associated with a higher risk of heart disease. Coconut oil, in contrast, is built from lauric and stearic acid. Early research shows that these fatty acids do not raise the risk of heart disease and may even have a beneficial effect on ratios of LDL and HDL. The effect of saturated plant fats on health has been studied in the context of various traditional diets. For example, Polynesians, who consume a diet rich in coconut milk, do not suffer widely from high cholesterol. Perhaps the building blocks in coconut fats combine to raise HDL. Or perhaps the effect of coconut fat may depend on whether you eat or do not eat a healthy diet. Based on the available facts, some scientists consider coconut oil to be a safe oil; others do not.

I do not use much coconut oil but I do use coconut milk fairly frequently, so I get my fair share of saturated coconut fats. My personal opinion is that saturated plant oils act differently in our bodies than saturated animal fats do. I believe that coconut oil is healthier for our bodies than butter. I think excess cholesterol which may result from too high an intake of animal fats interferes with how we process our omega-3 and -6 fats, but that reasonable amounts of saturated plant fats do not. I am convinced that environmental toxins concentrated in animal fats are part of the problem.

I also believe that how a specific food affects us depends on the amount of that food in the diet as well as how healthy the diet is overall. I believe that our bodies can thrive on reasonable amounts of unrefined saturated plant fats in the context of a good diet and that these are better for us than refined and processed vegetable oils. I also think that butter is preferable to refined, deodorized, and processed vegetable oils. Compared to coconut oil, however, butter is much higher on the food chain and brings with it greater amounts of persistent toxins and fatty acids that are hard on our bodies.

Ultimately, you will have to reach your own conclusion on the wisdom of eating coconut oil and coconut milk. If your physician recommends against coconut oil, you will manage just fine on the plan by respecting that advice and avoiding coconut fat. Alternatively, you might ask that you be allowed to try using coconut oil and see how it affects your general health and laboratory values.

ARE THE SATURATED FATS IN EGGS A PROBLEM?

The wisdom of including eggs in the diet raises as many questions as does coconut oil. Many people have been advised either to limit, or eliminate, egg yolks from their diet. I believe that fresh, whole eggs from a well-raised chicken are unlikely to cause any health problems.

Again, the jury is out on this question. There are studies showing that some people are "egg sensitive" in the sense that eggs adversely affect their blood fat ratios. There are good reasons to limit the presence of animal products in our diet and certainly we should be very concerned with the quality of the food we are eating. Many people are opting to avoid egg yolks and instead buy packaged egg whites from factory-farmed chickens. Is this a wise move? My opinion is no, it is not. Better to eat a few locally raised eggs than to buy cartons of egg whites laid by factory-farmed chickens and then pasteurized, preserved, and packaged for our use. But I know of no studies studying the health effect of eating fresh, local eggs compared to consuming commercial egg whites of unknown age and quality.

I also think there is an enormous difference between eating eggs from a healthy, reasonably content chicken and eating supermarket-quality eggs from factory-farmed chickens—even if those chickens are raised organically. The quality of feed and the stress generated by poor living conditions affect the ultimate healthfulness of the egg. If properly raised eggs from local chickens are not an option for you, you should look for a humane-certified source of supermarket eggs. Your best choice would then be organic eggs (those chickens are not fed genetically modified, sprayed grains), high in omega-3 fats (those chickens are fed foods high in omega-3 fats such as flax), and certified humane (meaning chickens have some room to move about, can take dust baths, and when the time comes are transported and slaughtered in a reasonably humane manner).

As with coconut oil, you have to make an individual decision about how eggs might affect your health. Again, perhaps your health care provider will allow you to try eating more eggs and then test to see how it affects your blood fat values. If not, there are many healthy breakfasts that can be made without eggs and there are many good substitutes for eggs in baking. Finally, of course, if you are allergic or hypersensitive to eggs, you should avoid them regardless of their effect on your blood fats.

Are safflower or sunflower oils healthy?

You may use any unrefined oil that is not deodorized, hydrogenated, or extracted using solvents, with the exception of canola, corn, cottonseed, non-organic soybean, and peanut oil. Safflower and sunflower oils are fine for limited use. However, both oils are high in omega-6 fats so neither should be used frequently. Be especially careful about eating chips. Most are composed of grains or high-glycemic vegetables high-heat cooked in either safflower or sunflower oils. These foods are not healthy; they are high in omega-6 fats, and are very easy to eat out of proportion. Sweet potato chips made with safflower oil may have more antioxidants than potatoes fried in canola oil but not by much. Both generate oxidative stress. Ultimately, chips are not fresh, whole foods and most often simply perpetuate cravings for empty calories. Crispy kale is a much healthier choice.

Questions about grains

Do we need grains in our diet?

Grains are optional on this plan; you may eliminate them entirely from your diet if you wish. This is radically different from government recommendations to eat more grains than fruits and vegetables, a recommendation that is built into many diet plans.

Whole grains contain fiber, a wide variety of phytonutrients, and vitamins, but do not contain anything that we cannot get from other plant foods that have been part of the human diet for a much longer period of time. Agriculture is relatively new and the grasses we now rely on so heavily (our grains) have not been part of our diet for very long. Grains caught on rapidly, however, as they are easily grown in poor soil, handle shorter summers, store well, and are filling. Grains quickly became a survival food for many and remain a survival food in many parts of the world today—for instance, rice is a grain that saves millions from starvation.

Most of us, however, have the luxury of being able to choose to thrive rather than simply survive. We do better without the sugars, omega-6 fats, and proteins such as gluten found in grains. We do better eating vegetables, nuts, and fruits. Those are foods we thrive on. But, because we have eaten grains since infancy, we often want them in our diet to sustain us emotionally—as a comfort food. Grains remain a choice to satisfy the need for comfort but, if you no longer crave them, you will do fine completely eliminating them or making them a special-occasion food.

Why do potatoes count as grain?

There is nothing inherently wrong with potatoes. They are a satisfying, tasty vegetable. The problem lies in our relationship with potatoes. Most Americans do not get anywhere near the recommended number of servings of fruits and vegetables each day, and of the servings they do eat, at least 40% are white potatoes. In other words, we favor potatoes out of proportion to their nutritional value and at the expense of getting the variety of vitamins, antioxidants, and other phytonutrients we need. Counting potato as a grain forces us to eat other fruits and vegetables and getting more variety is critical if we are to quiet inflammation.

Potatoes do have a high-glycemic index which means they can cause spikes in our blood sugar levels, triggering a greater release of insulin. Counting them as grains ensures that we eat other foods with them that will help moderate our blood sugar response.

Why are sprouted wheat tortillas not allowed?

When wheat is sprouted, some, but not all, of the gluten is transformed. Because so many people are extremely sensitive to gluten, it is important to eliminate all gluten during the Elimination Phase. As a result, we eliminate sprouted wheat until we are certain we are not wheat sensitive.

When corn is sprouted, some, but not all, of the protein that can cause a reaction is transformed. Because corn sensitivities are uncommon, most of us can eat sprouted corn. However, if it turns out that you are corn sensitive, you will need to give up sprouted corn tortillas and fresh corn as well.

QUESTIONS ABOUT SEAFOOD

WHY ARE FARMED SHELLFISH ALLOWED?

Most farmed shellfish (such as oysters, mussels, and clams) are not fed commercial feed. Even farmed varieties simply filter food from the water and therefore are not contaminated with antibiotics, drugs, rendered byproducts, and other ingredients typically fed to farmed fish. Farmed varieties of shellfish do not pose the problems that farmed fish do because they are eating their natural diet.

MAY I EAT TUNA FISH?

No. The Elimination Phase limits your choices to the seafood on the approved list. The approved wild fish are both sustainable and reasonably low in mercury, PCBs, and flame retardants. Most tuna comes from large species that are high on the food chain and have accumulated significant amounts of mercury and other toxins. Occasionally, you may come across small species of tuna, such as skipjack tuna caught with lines. That is the only tuna permitted as an everyday food after the Elimination and Testing Phases, but this tuna is difficult to find and much more expensive.

People often eat canned tuna in tuna salad where the tuna is mixed with onions, mayonnaise, pickles, and other ingredients. Canned wild salmon is easily substituted for the tuna in this type of salad with few people actually able to tell the difference. Those who can, usually find the salmon salad tastier. Sushi tuna is usually very high in mercury and should be avoided except as a special-occasion food after the Elimination and Testing Phases.

MAY I EAT SUSHI?

Most sushi is made with refined white rice to which sugar and rice wine have been added. Sushi and sashimi tuna usually tests very high in mercury and thus should be saved for special occasions even after the Elimination and Testing Phases. Some sushi bars offer sushi made with interesting vegetables such as wild carrot, burdock, shiitake, etc. instead of fish and use brown rice. You can also make healthy and delicious sushi using brown, black, or red rice without added sweeteners, and seafood on the approved list or any vegetables you choose. These types of sushi are allowed as long as the proportions are maintained by adding, for example, a seaweed salad to balance the rice.

May i eat smoked salmon?

Most smoked salmon (and other smoked fish) have added sugar and may not be eaten as an everyday food. However, some high-end restaurants and private fishermen smoke their own fish without adding sugar or other sweeteners. That type of smoked fish is fine and counts as protein in the proportionate meal.

Why is Alaskan halibut unsustainable?

I am not a fisheries expert. The information on the sustainability of the various species of seafood, and how polluted they are, comes from two sources: The Monterey Bay Aquarium (http://www.montereybayaquarium.org/cr/seafoodwatch.aspx) and Blue Ocean (http://www.blueocean.org/seafood/). Both manage very good websites and both will help you fine-tune your seafood list to suit you, your health needs, and the needs of the environment. When in doubt, contact them. This is especially important as the information on which species are sustainable may change over time. Do not follow them blindly, however. Increasingly they recommend some farmed fish in part to relieve the pressure consumers of placing on some wild fish. These groups do not always place as great a value on how healthy these fish may be for us.

Questions about beverages

Are there recommended amounts of water we should drink?

The plan does not recommend drinking any specific amount of water each day. On a typical Western diet, we eat little fresh fruit and vegetables. Most of our foods are dry and come in packets and boxes. These foods are high in salt, sugar, and chemicals. We need increased amounts of fluids to balance and flush those compounds out of our bodies.

When you adopt the Rule of Proportions and avoid added sugars and chemicals, your fluid intake from food rises (because you are eating water-filled fruits and vegetables) and your fluid needs decrease (because there are fewer compounds that need to be flushed out of your body). Most people do just fine drinking as

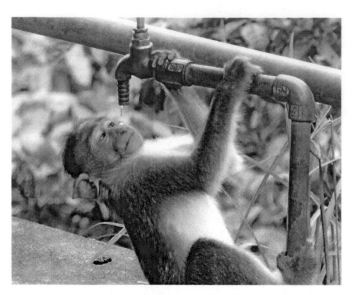

Let your thirst dictate how much you drink

much water as their thirst dictates. Of course, when in doubt drink a bit more water, especially if you are out in the sun where you may become dehydrated without noticing. Certainly, if you have a tendency to have muscle cramps or if you take a fiber supplement, you need to make sure you are drinking enough fluids.

What may i use to "doctor" my coffee and tea?

Coffee and tea contain caffeine and, although allowed, are not health foods. Often, people want to continue drinking them but actually do not like the way they taste. Instead, they want to both sweeten and "whiten" them to reduce the bitterness and to bind tannins in the beverages.

The rule is no added sweeteners of any kind. There is nothing you may add to sweeten these drinks. That said, people report being able to tolerate these beverages without added dairy by:

1. Switching to a different roast or a different variety. What you are drinking may be made much more palatable if you try a milder roast, a milder variety, or a higher-quality product.

2. Adding cinnamon or cardamom to coffee or tea. Strong Turkish coffee, for instance, is often brewed with spices as are many teas, known as chai.

3. Adding small amounts of coconut milk, nut milk, or unsweetened soy milk to beverages at meals and snacks. Do not drink "doctored" beverages between meals and snacks.

4. Most recommended is to learn to like the things you eat and drink. Many grow to enjoy (and even prefer) black coffee. Some discover that they manage quite well without these beverages and really do not like them except as vehicles for sugar and milk.

IS NON-DAIRY KEFIR ALLOWED ON THE PLAN?

Non-dairy kefir can be made from soy milk or the milk of nuts, seeds, coconut, or cereal grains. Yet another non-dairy kefir is made with sugar water mixed with citrus and dried fruit. This latter fizzy beverage is called "water kefir" and is prepared with a special variety of kefir grains called "sugary grains." Kefirs made from "not-milks" or from non–wheat related grains are fine provided they are not used in large amounts (they do not contain fiber), and provided they are eaten slowly with a spoon. Remember, we are trying not to drink our food. Water kefir is too sweet and is not allowed.

IS KOMBUCHA ALLOWED ON THE PLAN?

Traditional kombucha is made from fermented black tea. Sugar is added but the yeast transform it in the fermentation process. The end product contains only a small amount of natural sugars, and it is fine to drink kombucha with meals. It is not allowed between meals and snacks because of its natural sugars. Other fruit-flavored kombuchas are not allowed. They are more akin to fruit juice as they contain too much sugar and no fiber.

WHAT CAUSES WINE AND ALCOHOL SENSITIVITIES?

Alcohol presents many problems for the body. This is why it is eliminated during the Elimination and Testing Phases.

Alcohol does not have to be digested; it is absorbed instantly into the body and is quickly found in all organs. It immediately decreases the production of a hormone that inhibits urination. Alcohol acts as a diuretic while at the same time increasing the release of magnesium in the urine. Dehydration is one problem with alcohol. Depletion of the mineral magnesium is another.

While the liver is breaking down alcohol, it stops maintaining our blood sugar and does not convert glycogen to glucose. This tends to make us a bit hypoglycemic, which increases the temptation to eat sugary, refined foods that increase, rather than relieve, inflammation.

In the first stage of alcohol detoxification, the liver uses dehydrogenase enzymes to break down the ethanol in the beverage. Many individuals lack adequate amounts of these enzymes and more rapidly feel the negative effects of alcohol. This is one reason for a hypersensitivity to alcohol, one that is particularly common in people of Asian or Jewish descent. Amounts of these enzymes also vary between ages, sexes, and individuals. For instance, young women generally have less than young men and do not process alcohol as efficiently. All alcohol contains small amounts of methanol that breaks down into formaldehyde and is processed once the ethanol in the drink has been broken down. Our reactions to the toxins generated in this process vary but they can add to our sensitivity to alcohol.

We may also be affected by congeners. Congeners are toxic chemicals that are formed during fermentation, and some types of alcohol have more of them than others. These congeners are widely deemed responsible for headaches associated with alcohol intake. Vodka has fewer congeners than gin. Most scotch whiskey has about four times more congeners than gin. Bourbon has about eight times as many as gin and nearly 30 times as many as vodka. Red wine has more congeners than white wine does. But any congeners at all may be too many for you.

Of course, as these metabolites, toxins, and chemicals build up and interfere with the usual functions of the liver, kidney, and brain, the body responds with inflammation, releasing cytokines that increase the malaise that many feel after drinking.

Wine affects histamine levels. It is often postulated that foods that contain histamine can result in symptoms similar to an allergic reaction. Furthermore, they can delay the metabolism of histamine, and increase the concentration of histamine in blood. In addition, the ethanol and acetaldehyde constituents of wine can stimulate the release of endogenous histamine. There is disagreement as to whether or not the histamine in wine is a problem, but it may be. If you think histamine may be a problem for you, you should test other foods that affect histamine levels such as sardines and anchovies, ripened cheeses, hard-cured sausages, fermented foods, chocolate, and bananas as well.

Sulfites in wine may also be a problem. Sulfites occur naturally and plants use them to prevent microbial growth. They are found on grapes, onions, garlic, and on many other plants. No wine can ever be "sulfite free" because they are on the grapes used to produce wine. Some vintners, however, add significantly more sulfites. The best way to test for a sulfite sensitivity is to eat a food high in natural sulfites—for instance, dried apricots. Two ounces of dried apricots will have 10 times more sulfites than a glass of wine. If you eat those apricots and have a reaction, you know sulfites in excess are a problem. If you do not, it could be a combination of *any* of the many factors described above that makes alcohol difficult for your body to process.

These various effects also explain why, when you do choose to drink alcohol, it should be done in moderation and in the context of a meal that helps quiet the inflammatory response the alcohol will trigger. Detoxifying vegetables combined with lots of water will help significantly. It is also important to understand that alcohol does place a burden on the body and, even in moderate amounts combined with antioxidant-rich foods, may cause you to plateau.

QUESTIONS ABOUT TOXINS AND TROUBLESOME COMPOUNDS
DO VEGETABLE WASHES FOR NON-ORGANIC PRODUCE HELP?

Vegetable washes remove pesticide residues from the surface of fruits and vegetables. This can reduce the amount of toxins on the food.

Today, however, many insecticides, herbicides, and fungicides are systemic. This means that they are absorbed into the plant itself. Washing will not reduce the amount of chemicals found in such foods. While there is no way to determine which chemicals are on any particular piece of food, it is nevertheless wise to wash conventional products with these types of soaps.

No, heterocyclic amines (HCAs) are formed from the condensation of creatinine with amino acids during the cooking of meat and animal products. Temperature, processing, cooking time, and the types of amino acid present affect the formation of these compounds. In general, cooking at higher temperatures and for longer periods of time increases the amount of HCAs. Frying or grilling of red meats produces more HCAs than do indirect heat methods such as stewing, steaming, and poaching.

Although some HCAs may be formed in smoking meat or fish, the concerns with wood-smoked food are different. Wood smoke contains at least a hundred polycyclic hydrocarbons and alkylated derivatives, many of which are carcinogenic. Benzo[a]pyrene is often used as a marker of carcinogenic compounds in smoke and smoked fish. Of course, it is possible to combine high heat, wood smoke, and red meat, in which case both HCAs and benzo[a]pyrene-type compounds would form, leading to a real problem food.

Foods high in either compound should not be eaten daily and, when eaten, should be combined with ample amounts of nutrient-dense vegetables. The proportionate meal ensures that this happens, but adding a little extra on the vegetable side would be a good idea when indulging in these foods.

HOW DID FLAME RETARDANTS COME TO ACCUMULATE IN FISH?

As one student pointed out, it is really ironic that fish are so high in flame retardants. Being surrounded by water, they are at extraordinarily low risk for catching on fire.

The pathway that leads flame retardants to accumulate in the environment remains a mystery. We do know that a typical American comes in contact with dozens, if not hundreds, of products that contain flame retardants every day, ranging from electronics, electrical cables, carpets, furniture, textiles to our food. Flame retardants are found worldwide in house dust, indoor and outdoor air, and the water and sediments of rivers, estuaries, and oceans. They are concentrated in whales, seals, birds, moose, deer, mussels, and probably all freshwater and marine fish.

And flame retardants are on the rise. In one five-year period the concentration of flame retardants found in halibut more than doubled while the amount in striped bass tripled. In a twenty-year period the amount of flame retardants found in the milk of Swedish mothers increased 55 times. The amount in U.S. mothers' milk is much higher than that of women elsewhere in the world. Nonetheless, most flame retardants remain virtually unregulated in this country and most of the world.

DO SEAWEEDS AND SEA VEGETABLES CONCENTRATE TOXINS?

First, let us look at the health benefits of seaweeds and sea vegetables: They are rich in trace minerals and interesting complex sugars. They reduce both blood pressure and serum cholesterol, and they have antibiotic and anti-tumor properties. They seem particularly good at preventing colon, rectal, and breast cancer, sarcoma, and leukemia. They appear to inhibit the herpes virus.

Seaweeds contain alginic acid, a polysaccharide, which binds with any heavy metals found in the intestines, and causes them to be eliminated. So, heavy metals, such as barium, cadmium, lead, mercury, zinc, and even radioactive strontium, that may be present in the intestines will not be absorbed by the body when sufficient alginic acid is present.

On the other hand, because sea vegetables are mineral accumulators, they will tend to concentrate heavy metals if grown and gathered in polluted places. It appears that much of the seaweed on the market today is farmed away from polluted areas (farming of seaweed appears sustainable at this point in time), and has not been shown to be a problem. It is recommended that you from time to time inquire where the sea vegetables you are using come from and to make sure that they continue to be sustainable. Unfortunately as I write this, radioactive material from the Fukushima nuclear plant is seeping and being dumped into the Pacific Ocean. It may be that we will have to avoid seaweed from previously "clean" harvesting areas.

CAN ORGANIC ANIMAL PRODUCTS BE FACTORY-FARMED?

Yes. There are many advantages to choosing certified organic animal products but the rules governing organic still leave much to be desired both from a health and a humane perspective. They are also in a constant state of flux. The rules governing organic feed inputs eliminate many types of feed that cause concern: Antibiotics, GM products, animal byproducts, artificial colors/flavors, synthetic flowing agents, and synthetic preservatives are not permitted in any organic feed products. There are rules requiring animals have better access to the out-of-doors, but these rules often fall short of what many wish: The USDA in 2010 passed new rules requiring organic dairy cows to be pastured at least 120 days of the growing season and that they must eat from the pasture at least 30% of the time.

The new rules also apply to cattle raised for beef. In the case of beef cattle, however, the requirement that 30 percent of food must come from pasture is lifted during the so-called finishing period, when the animals are being fattened for slaughter and are often fed grain. During that period they must still be allowed to graze, however.

In the end, the answer is that organic standards do not preclude factory farming nor are they perfect. The quality of animal products varies from one farm to another. Thus, you should always contact the farm to make sure that it is raising animals in a way that mirrors your expectations for a healthy food product.

HOW IS HIGH-FRUCTOSE CORN SYRUP DIFFERENT FROM CORN SYRUP?

Corn syrup is prepared through a series of chemical steps. First, corn is soaked in hot water and sulfur dioxide. Corn starch is then separated out from this slurry. The starch is made up of chains of sugars, and a variety of chemicals are used to break them into shorter chains. Corn syrup is made up of short chains that are quite sweet. High-fructose corn syrup (HFCS), which is sweeter than regular corn syrup, is made through an enzymatic process that converts the glucose in corn syrup into fructose. It is then back-blended with pure glucose to achieve the desired sweetness. Often, contaminated caustic soda and hydrochloric acid are used in this process and carry mercury as a contaminant into the final end product.

Neither corn syrup nor HFCS occur naturally. The Center for Science in the Public Interest argues that, because of the high level of processing and the use of at least one genetically modified (GM) enzyme in making of HFCS, it is wrong to call it "natural."

One study found that soft drinks sweetened with HFCS have up to ten times the amount of harmful carbonyl compounds compared to other sugar-sweetened soft drinks. These carbonyl compounds are blamed for causing diabetic complications such as foot ulcers and eye and nerve damage.

Honeybees in the U.S. are increasingly fed HFCS instead of fructose. One study showed that, at certain temperatures, HFCS rapidly begins to form a compound that is toxic to honeybees.

There is an ongoing debate between various scientists and the corn industry about the healthfulness (or lack thereof) of these corn sweeteners. More information is available at sites such as http://en.wikipedia.org/wiki/High-fructose_corn_syrup.

This plan simply eliminates them in favor of healthy foods.

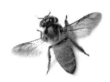

PART THREE
The Testing Phase

CHAPTER TWENTY-TWO

Food Sensitivity Testing

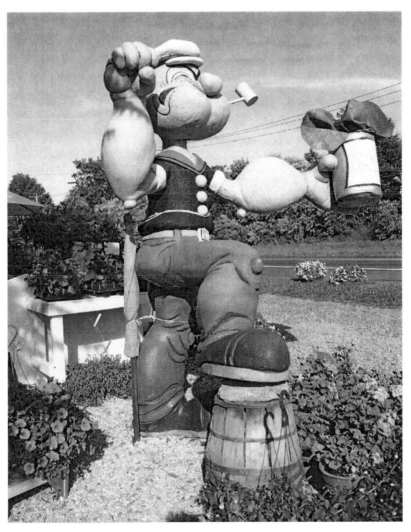

Making sure the foods we eat work for us

At the end of three weeks on the Elimination Phase, you should be feeling much better. You will have begun to lose weight (if needed) and/or reduce your aches and pains. If so, you are ready to begin testing for food sensitivities. However, if you have not experienced much improvement, you should read the chapter on Troublesome Plateaus before reading this chapter and testing any foods.

We can react negatively to any food in several ways: The most severe reaction is a true food allergy where the body forms a permanent antibody memory against a compound in a specific food. Food allergies may be severe and build to anaphylactic shock (which can be fatal). It is critical that people with true food allergies strictly and completely avoid foods they are allergic to. Laboratory tests can accurately detect food allergies.

In the case of a food sensitivity, the immune system becomes highly "suspicious" of a food compound, usually because a complex part of a food molecule has crossed the intestinal barrier and entered the body proper. The immune system perceives this molecule as foreign and reacts to other "foreigners" present in the digestive system by attracting additional immune cells to prepare for a potential invasion. This inflammatory response recurs every time we eat a "suspect" food.

Food sensitivities do not cause immediate and ever stronger reactions the way food allergies do. In fact, people with one or more food sensitivities often do not know that a specific food is causing inflammation. The symptoms of a food sensitivity can be highly variable. Depending on the individual's cytokine imbalance, the symptoms can vary from postnasal drip to headaches to indigestion to joint aches and more.

Unlike food allergies, there are no completely reliable laboratory tests for food sensitivities. These inflammatory immune responses can, however, be detected by elimination/reintroduction testing.[1] During the Elimination Phase, we eliminated four foods that commonly trigger reactions: Wheat, dairy, peanuts, and dried corn. To test them, we reintroduce them one by one to see if we react.

As we test these four foods, we ask ourselves how nutritious the food feels. Each of these four foods has some negative aspects that are summarized in the sections titled "Cautionary Comments." Thinking about how we feel when we reintroduce a food will help us decide how we want to fit the food into our daily diet if we are not sensitive to it.

KEYS TO SENSITIVITY TESTING

1. To test a food, we need to reduce overall inflammation by staying on the Elimination Phase for at least three weeks. In order to "hear" if a food is inflammatory, background "inflammatory noise" caused by intestinal flora imbalances, too much oxidative stress, too many omega-6 fats, and so on must be quieted. If you have had wine or sugar or made other exceptions during the Elimination Phase on more than at most two or three occasions, you need to wait until you have three almost perfect weeks under your belt before you begin testing.

2. You must not have eaten any of the foods you are about to test in the week prior (preferably three weeks prior) to testing. If you had a piece of bread a few days ago or some milk in your coffee, put off testing until at least seven days have elapsed since you ate them.

3. You must eat a substantial amount of the test food for the number of days indicated in the instructions. As a rule, you cannot conclude that you are not sensitive by adding back a small amount of a suspect food. Having a few pieces of toast or some cheese will not necessarily cause a perceptible inflammatory response. Most of us would rather not know that we are sensitive to a food that we enjoy eating, so we avoid unwanted results by only eating a little of a suspect food and declaring that it did not cause a reaction. Remember, testing is meant to be a journey of discovery; learning

---

[1] Note that this type of testing is inappropriate for food allergies. In cases of true food allergies, the problem food should never be eaten.

that you are sensitive to a food does not mean that you have to avoid that food for all time, so do not fudge the test results.

4. Do not attempt to explain away any symptoms you experience. Record everything. It is important to fight any tendency to ignore mild symptoms. One example is the person who reports, "I ate a piece of toast and I felt a little congested, but I am fighting off a cold and I do not think I reacted to wheat." Instead, assume the congestion is a food reaction. If you are skeptical about the results, you should retest the food.

5. Some people have an immediate and strong reaction to even a small amount of a reintroduced food. This can occur in response to a food they have previously eaten on a regular basis without any problems at all. If you experience a strong reaction to a food, you should discontinue the test as soon as you react.

6. Although rare, reactions may be delayed up to 48 hours after you last ate the food, so include any reactions you experience in the 48 hours after you stop eating a test food.[2]

TESTING WHEAT, A TWO-DAY TEST

1. Wheat is a grain and may be eaten for lunch, dinner, and both snacks. It should, however, not be eaten at breakfast. Try to eat some form of wheat at both snacks, lunch, and dinner for two days. The more wheat you eat, the more accurate the test will be.

2. At a minimum, eat wheat three times a day. You are trying to evaluate how your body handles a group of wheat proteins (called gluten). If you only eat a small amount, the background inflammation in your body may mask a gluten sensitivity. Record any reactions on the chart on page 252.

3. Remember proportions while testing: A maximum of one-third of a meal or snack may consist of wheat because it is a grain.

4. Wheat products should be labeled whole wheat, not whole grain because, by law, whole grain products need only contain 51%

---

[2] This is rare so you may choose not to wait 48 hours in between tests. However, if you are among the few who do have delayed reactions, you will blame your symptoms on the "wrong" food. This is, however, easily revealed when you add that food back into your regular diet and it makes you feel worse.

whole grain. These "whole grain" breads often contain 49% white, refined flour which is inflammatory and should not be tested.[3]

5. Avoid any bread that is squishy. Squishy breads typically contain refined flour, dough conditioners, and other chemicals. Look for dense, heavy, whole wheat bread, wheat berries, whole wheat pasta, spelt products, or whole wheat tortillas. Again, keep in mind the recommended proportions of grains to vegetables and fruit.

6. Breads may have some sugar or other sweetener on the ingredient list but the sweetener should appear as one of the last ingredients. In that case, the sugar was used to feed the yeast and help the bread rise. If the sugar is one of the first ingredients, it was added to make the bread taste sweeter; such breads need to be avoided during testing.

7. Eat primarily the following forms of wheat: Bulgur, kamut, seitan[4] (wheat gluten), spelt, triticale, wheat berries, wheat bran, wheat germ, and whole wheat. Some, but only a few test meals, may include the wheat relatives: Rye, barley, and oats. These wheat relatives may not trigger a reaction in wheat-sensitive people, even though wheat would.

8. Sprouted wheat products should not be used as test foods. Sprouting converts much of the gluten in wheat, making it difficult to gauge how your body handles gluten.

9. At the end of the two days, quit eating wheat. Wait two days or until any symptoms have resolved (this sometimes takes longer than two days) before testing the next food. Do not eat any wheat while testing other foods, even if you do not test positive for a wheat sensitivity.

---

[3] Alternatively, you may contact manufacturers of whole grain foods to learn if they actually are made entirely from whole wheat and contain no refined flour.

[4] Seitan is available in the refrigerated dairy section of most grocery stores. It usually is chicken- or beef-flavored and is used as a meat substitute. Seitan is a common ingredient in many vegetarian dishes served at Chinese restaurants. Because it is pure wheat gluten, it is an ideal test food.

CAUTIONARY COMMENTS ON WHEAT

Wheat and other grains are relatively new foods in the human diet. Before agriculture, our ancestors lived as hunter/gatherers. Plants dispersed their seed as far away from the parent plant as possible. Some plants used the wind to carry off the seed. Some relied on birds or other animals to eat their fruits and disperse the seeds. Other plants developed seed heads that shattered and spread the seeds.

Plants did not typically hold their seeds neatly on seed heads as, for instance, corn does today. Seeds were more difficult to gather, and humans did not eat much grain seed. Only with the advent of agriculture and the gradual selection of plants that held their seeds tightly—making harvesting grain much easier—did humans begin to eat much grain. There are many indications that our bodies have not had time to adapt well to eating large quantities of grain.

Grains are an inexpensive food that allowed many people, especially the poor, to subsist and survive. Grains are easy to grow and store, and they are filling. Thus, while not necessarily an optimal food, they quickly became a prominent part of the human diet. Grains easily become comfort foods because they provide sugars, which our bodies crave, and because they are foods we enjoyed as children.

Because they are seeds, grains are higher in omega-6 fats. In our culture, we have to continually work on getting enough omega-3 fats to balance our omega-6s. The less grain we eat, the easier it is to achieve and maintain a healthy omega-6:3 ratio.

Wheat contains gluten and gluten is inflammatory to a significant portion of the population. It is a very common cause of food sensitivities. In addition, there are indications that even people without any noticeable sensitivity to wheat produce more inflammatory cytokines after eating wheat. This has caused some commentators to ask whether anyone should eat wheat on a regular basis.

Finally, studies indicate that people who eat grains for breakfast typically experience more food cravings later on in the day than those who eat protein in the morning. Thus, eating grains appears to make it more difficult to maintain steady glucose levels which, in turn, makes healthy eating more difficult.

There is a place in the proportionate meal for those who wish to eat whole grains because they do provide fiber and other healthy plant constituents. Nonetheless, grains could be entirely omitted from our diet without causing any adverse health effects. As you test wheat, consider how much of your plate your body (as opposed to your mind) would like to see filled with wheat. Many people end up deciding to have wheat only as a special-occasion food (see chapter 24) because they discover that other foods make them feel better and are more satisfying.

Testing dairy, a three-day test

1. Add dairy back into your diet, eating as much dairy as you can for three days, keeping proportions in mind. You are trying to evaluate how your body handles a group of milk proteins.

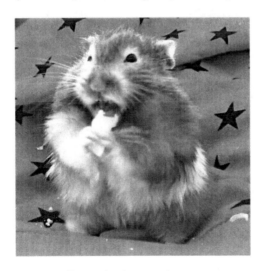

Szarotka loves cheese

If you only eat a small amount, the background inflammation in your body may mask your dairy sensitivity. Record any reactions on the chart on page 252.

2. Dairy is a protein and you may have dairy at all three meals and both snacks. It should not, however, make up more than one-half of your breakfast or one-third of any other meal or snack.

3. If your dairy is organic, you avoid antibiotics, synthetic bovine growth hormones, animals fed genetically modified grain, etc. If possible, eat dairy products from grass-fed and grass-finished cows for an improved omega-6:3 ratio.

4. Avoid cheeses containing dyes, stabilizers, or other chemicals.

5. Any yoghurt you eat must be unsweetened and without honey, jam, or other added sweeteners. You may, however, add cut-up fruit.

6. To test, you should eat cheese, cottage cheese, cream cheese, milk, and yoghurt. You may add small amounts of butter, ghee, and sour cream for flavor while you are testing dairy but you may not cook in them—olive oil must remain the primary fat in your diet.[5] Dairy sensitivities are reactions to proteins in dairy. Butter, ghee, and sour cream are fats with only small amounts of protein and cannot be relied on to measure a sensitivity to dairy proteins.

7. Focus on testing dairy products from cows. A few of your meals or snacks may be goat or sheep products, but most should be cow dairy.

8. We test dairy for three days, a day longer than wheat, because dairy is frequently consumed either as yoghurt or as cheese. While yoghurt contains the same proteins as milk—and may cause the same immune response—the beneficial bacteria present in the yoghurt tends to mask our reactions to it. Cheese is typically mostly fat, and thus lower in the sensitizing proteins. This too may mask our reaction to dairy.

9. If you are lactose-intolerant, take lactaid, or test only lactose-free dairy products.

Record your reactions on the chart on page 252. At the end of three days, after eating ample amounts of dairy, quit eating dairy. Wait until any symptoms have resolved before moving on to test the next food. Do not eat dairy again, even if you did not react negatively, until all of the suspect foods have been tested.

---

[5] Thus, you may add a pat of butter to a baked potato but you may not cook your food in butter instead of olive oil. Nor should you make butter-based sauces.

CAUTIONARY COMMENTS ON DAIRY

Our hunter/gatherer ancestors lived in a time before cows were domesticated; they did not eat cheese or drink milk. After being weaned, they most likely drank only water or water infused with herbs or chunks of food (e.g., soups or stews). The idea of confining animals, removing the baby animals from their mothers, and appropriating their milk is a relatively new concept. We have not had much time to adapt to dairy and many do not thrive on it.

Dairy in any form is a concentrated source of animal protein, milk sugar, and fats. Given how most dairy cows are fed and raised today, the fats consist mostly of cholesterol and omega-6 fats. In addition, because cows are high on the food chain, dairy fat contains persistent environmental toxins such as DDT, PCBs, perfluorinated chemicals, radioactive iodine and cesium, etc. (see chapter 8). This is true even for organic, pasture-raised animals.

Excess animal protein burdens the liver, the kidneys, and the bones (see chapter 16). Research suggests that, while milk contains a significant amount of calcium, dairy products are not the best source of calcium for our bodies because dairy feeds microbes that make us less able to absorb calcium. Eating kale and other green vegetables may be a better source because their calcium is better absorbed. In addition, there are strong indications that we actually excrete more calcium than we absorb when we eat dairy products. If this is true, and it well may be, then dairy is actually a poor source of calcium.

While there is room on the proportionate plate for dairy, many people choose to make dairy a special-occasion food rather than eating it daily.

TESTING PEANUTS, A ONE-DAY TEST

1. Peanuts count as protein and you include them in all your test meals and snacks as this is only a one-day test. Peanuts should not, however, make up more than one-half of breakfast or one-third of other meals or snacks. At the end of the day, stop eating peanuts and wait until any symptoms have resolved before moving on to test the next food. Again, exclude peanuts while testing other foods, even in the absence of any signs of a sensitivity.

CAUTIONARY COMMENTS ABOUT PEANUTS

Many people in North America are extremely allergic to peanuts. Peanut allergies are not as common in countries where fewer peanuts are consumed. While some people are sensitive (as opposed to allergic) to peanuts, this is very uncommon. However, peanuts are quite susceptible to molds and many people react to molds. Thus, molds may periodically, and somewhat erratically, cause inflammatory responses that are blamed on the peanuts.

One of the molds that grows on peanuts is *Aspergillus flavus*. This mold produces aflatoxin B, a very strong liver carcinogen.

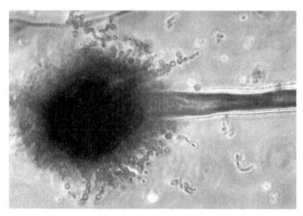

Aspergillus flavus a dangerous mold

Aflatoxin continues to be formed by the mold after peanuts are harvested. To slow the production of this toxin, always refrigerate peanuts and peanut butter once the jar is opened.

Because peanuts are so susceptible to molds, there is a reasonable basis for concern that organic peanuts may carry more molds. However, buying commercial peanuts is not a satisfactory solution. Non-organic peanuts still often test positive for aflatoxin, but are also typically treated with highly toxic fungicides.

Ultimately, the main reason we eliminated peanuts was to encourage us to eat other wholesome, tasty nuts and nut butters besides peanuts. Walnuts, for instance, are high in omega-3 oils and make a tasty snack and oil. Almonds make a delicious nut butter. Peanuts are relatively easy to replace in our diet, reducing our exposure to molds and chemicals.

TESTING DRIED CORN, A ONE-DAY TEST

1. Eat ample amounts of dried corn in the form of polenta, grits, popcorn, corn chips, tortillas, and cereals for a one-day test. You may want to eat more fresh and sprouted corn at the same time to measure the full effect of corn in your diet. Record any reactions on the chart on page 253.
2. Corn is a grain and should be eaten for both snacks, lunch, and dinner but not for breakfast. Treat dried corn as grain in terms of serving size.
3. Do not add back foods containing high-fructose corn syrup or other corn chemicals.
4. Much of the dried corn comes from genetically modified seed. You avoid GM seed by only eating organic dried corn foods.
5. Do not eat popcorn or corn chips without fruits or vegetables. Crispy kale is a good food to have with popcorn (to make it easier to eat proportionately) or better, instead of popcorn. Have your own bowl of guacamole or salsa so you can double or triple dip your chips.
6. At the end of the day, remove corn from your diet. Wait for any symptoms to resolve before testing any additional foods. Do not eat dried corn again until you are done testing.

CAUTIONARY COMMENTS ON EATING CORN

Corn is a seed and a higher omega-6 food. We can enjoy fresh corn, a tasty sweet vegetable, as long as we also eat a variety of other vegetables. Dried corn is more problematic because much of the dried corn crop is genetically modified (see chapter 20). Also, corn has become a prominent component of most processed food, either as corn derivatives that are part corn and part chemical such as dextrose, maltodextrin, modified corn starch, corn syrups, etc. or as corn oil, a high omega-6 oil present in many processed foods. Eliminating dried corn from the everyday diet eliminates the temptation to eat foods containing these problematic ingredients.

Corn is also very prone to *Aspergillus flavus* (see cautionary comments about peanuts), a very troublesome mold. But the biggest problem with dried corn is that our favorite corn products are difficult to eat proportionately. It is hard to eat two handfuls of fruit for every handful of popcorn. It is hard to fit twice as much dip on a single chip and it is very easy to eat chips alone. Many people ultimately decide that they are quite happy with sprouted corn tortillas as an everyday food and only occasionally eat polenta or corn bread in a context where proportions can be maintained. Many find that a bowl of crispy kale is as satisfying as a bowl of popcorn and, unlike popcorn, can be eaten by itself making proportions easy to maintain.

RECORDING SYMPTOMS OF FOOD SENSITIVITIES

It is very important to acknowledge symptoms that occur when you are testing a food. Remember, if you answer "yes" to any question on the chart while testing a food, you should assume that you are sensitive to the suspect food.

Read over the list of common symptoms on the charts at the end of this chapter frequently while testing, and monitor your responses carefully. Do not "explain away" any response, even a mild response. Any symptoms, even mild ones, suggest that the food is increasing inflammation in your body. If you doubt a result, you should retest that food after staying on the Elimination Phase for another seven or more days.

SENSITIVITIES AND FOOD CRAVINGS

Foods change our body chemistry. Sometimes, when we eat an inflammatory food, we may enjoy some of the chemical changes that result. The rush of energy we experience then causes us to want to eat more and more of that food. While we fully intended just to have a single piece of bread, we find ourselves heading back to the kitchen for more until the loaf is gone. Lack of moderation is a symptom of a food sensitivity. People simply do not experience broccoli and other green vegetables as irresistible and many a head of cabbage or cauliflower has sat quietly in the fridge without calling out anyone's name. In contrast, bread and cheese are often difficult to eat in moderation.

Other times, we may dislike the chemical changes a particular food causes when we eat it. Many of us then begin craving different foods, for example, sugar, refined grains, or fats. This new craving is an attempt to self-medicate away the discomfort the food caused. Thus, a person plans to have a slice of bread and has no problems putting away the loaf of bread after eating a slice. But, because the bread causes uncomfortable biochemical sensations, soon the person experiences an irresistible craving for a candy bar despite having gone weeks without any sugar cravings. We often turn to sweet, fatty foods to make us feel better (this tactic, unfortunately, does not work well, see p. 168.) In many cases, difficult sugar cravings are caused by a person continually eating an inflammatory food rather than a lack of willpower or a sugar addiction *per se*.

The importance of food sensitivities

It is important to acknowledge any food sensitivities you may have. Food sensitivities are important because they directly trigger inflammation. Unlike oxidative stress that can be quieted with antioxidants, an engaged immune system is difficult to calm down. Continuously eating foods that our immune system thinks are dangerous will have an adverse effect on our health—and weight—even if we are eating only small amounts that seemingly produce only negligible symptoms.

A splash of milk in your coffee will trigger the release of inflammatory cytokines and inflammation even if you do not perceive much of a reaction. If you are sensitive to a food, it is very important to quit eating that food regularly. It should not be part of your daily diet, even in very small amounts. While we should not regularly eat foods that we are sensitive to, this does not mean that we must avoid that food at all times. We can cope with things that are not optimal as long as we only do so occasionally. Thus, we may be dairy sensitive and have to give up milk in our coffee on a daily basis. We will still be able to have a caffe latte or ice cream for dessert for special occasions (see chapter 24).

Retesting suspect foods

Sometimes people do not believe that their mild symptoms—for instance, congestion—were caused by the test food. Retesting is then in order to clarify whether there is a sensitivity.

More often, individuals will want to know if they are sensitive to an entire food group. For instance, it is possible to be sensitive to one of the gluten proteins in wheat but not react to rye or oat proteins, even though some of their proteins resemble gluten. A person may react to cow dairy but may be fine with goat or sheep products. Retesting is appropriate in all these cases.

To retest, stay on the Elimination Phase for an additional week. Then retest the suspect food. In other words:

If you question the results of the first test, retest wheat for two days or retest dairy for three days.

If you want to know if you can tolerate a related food, test rye and/or oats for two days (omitting all wheat) or test sheep and goat dairy products for three days (omitting all cow dairy).

Again, it is important to eat a significant amount of any food you are testing. It will not suffice to have a small serving of goat yoghurt and a little goat cheese.

FREQUENTLY ASKED QUESTIONS RE: TESTING

Q: Do I have to test now? I am just settling into the Elimination Phase and do not want to add any foods back just yet. Do I have to?

A: No. The Elimination Phase is optimally healthy and you may eat that way for the rest of your life if you wish.

Q: When is the best time to test for food sensitivities?

A: It is important to test for them before inflammatory foods begin reappearing in your life.

During the Elimination Phase we carefully avoid inflammatory foods and do not consume sugar, refined flour, chemicals, or alcohol. We are precise about proportions and eat large amounts of fruits and vegetables. Eventually we may begin to deviate from the Elimination Phase rules from time to time. It is important to test for food sensitivities before inflammatory foods begin reappearing in our lives because we need to be in a quieted state to effectively test for sensitivities. Unfortunately, those who delay testing often begin to make exceptions. With those exceptions—a glass of wine now and again, some desserts (often a combination of sugar, wheat, and dairy), more saturated animal fats, less precise proportions—inflammation increases. If we test a food in this more inflamed state, we may incorrectly conclude that we are not sensitive to a food because the food does not make us feel much worse than we already do.

It is important to test for food sensitivities before making exceptions to the Elimination Phase. If you decide to put off testing for a while, make sure you begin testing at once if you find yourself tempted to deviate from the rules. Remember, you can test a food and then eliminate it again for as long as you wish. Testing does not have to be synonymous with adding test foods back into your eating plan.

Q: I know I am sensitive to one of the foods; should I test it?

A: Possibly. If you know, for instance, that you are sensitive to dairy, you may wish to test or retest it to see if your body still reacts to it. However, only do this if you have avoided consuming dairy for six months or more. If you have not eliminated it for that long there is no need to inflame your body by testing it again.

Q: If I find I am sensitive to a food during testing, does this mean I will always be sensitive to it?

A: No, if you eliminate a food you are sensitive to for a prolonged period (six months or more) and eat properly, you may heal your intestinal lining and give your immune system time to "forget" that a food seems dangerous. You may at some point overcome your food sensitivity as well as reduce any seasonal allergies you may have. So, many months down the road you may want to go back on the Elimination Phase and retest those foods again. Note, however, you should never test foods that you have a true allergy to; those will not diminish over time.

Q: May I vary the order of testing? I really would like to eat dairy again as soon as possible?

A: Yes, you may test these foods in any order you wish. You may also wait longer in between testing foods—as long as you remain on the Elimination Phase. That is, you may begin by testing dairy one week. A week later, you may opt to test corn. Yet a week later, you may opt to test wheat. This is fine, as long as you do not start having sugar and other inflammatory foods that will impair your ability to test your reactions.

Testing Wheat and Dairy		
Symptom	Wheat	Dairy
Nasal congestion		
Chest congestion		
Headaches		
Brain fog or mood changes		
Joint aches		
Muscle aches		
Pain		
Fatigue		
Poor sleep		
Circles under eyes		
Changes in body odor		
Changes in skin (e.g., acne, rashes, itching)		
Changes in bowel function or digestion		
Can you eat this food in moderation or is it a trigger food for you?		
Did your food cravings change?		
Does this feel like a nutritious food?		
Other negative changes?		

Testing Corn and Peanuts		
Symptom	Corn	Peanuts
Nasal congestion		
Chest congestion		
Headaches		
Brain fog or mood changes		
Joint aches		
Muscle aches		
Pain		
Fatigue		
Poor sleep		
Circles under eyes		
Changes in body odor		
Changes in skin (e.g., acne, rashes, itching)		
Changes in bowel function or digestion		
Can you eat this food in moderation or is it a trigger food for you?		
Did your food cravings change?		
Does this feel like a nutritious food?		
Other negative changes?		

CHAPTER TWENTY-THREE
Troublesome Plateaus

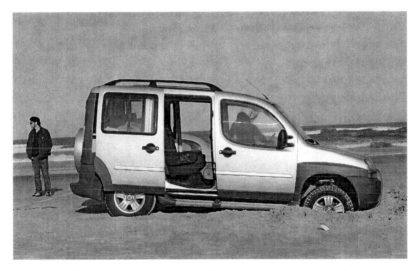

Feeling stuck and unable to make progress?

After three weeks on the Elimination Phase, some people will neither have lost weight nor experienced much improvement in any symptoms. Others may initially lose inches and start to feel better but then improvement slows or stops. People in the second group feel somewhat better but significant symptoms of inflammation may remain. We refer to this as a plateau. Plateaus can be overcome but to do so requires a bit of soul-searching, investigation, and discipline. It is, however, incredibly important to do this work in order to quiet inflammation.

The first step in evaluating a plateau is to look carefully at what and when you are eating.

1. ARE YOU TRULY CLOSELY FOLLOWING THE PLAN?

Make sure that:

- You are not eating grain for breakfast.

- You are eating some protein with fruit and/or vegetables soon after you get up.

- You are not grazing between meals and snacks, and are not eating two to three hours before bedtime.

- You are eating proportionate meals. At least two-thirds of every lunch, dinner, and snack consists of vegetables and fruit with an emphasis on green vegetables rather than fruit.

- You have not indulged in refined grain, sugar, fatty meats, or alcohol on more than one or at most two occasions during the three-week Elimination Phase.

2. ARE YOU EATING ENOUGH GREEN VEGETABLES?

Green vegetables are our greatest allies in quieting inflammation. Fruits and root vegetables have lots of antioxidants, fiber, and vitamins. They are important in our diet but to make significant progress, we need to substantially increase our intake of green vegetables. Look over your eating patterns for the last week or two. Are you primarily eating fruit and sweeter vegetables such as carrots, potatoes, beets, corn, and tomatoes? If so, you may notice enormous positive change if you instead eat green vegetables at least twice a day, including a significant amount of dark, leafy greens and cruciferous vegetables.

3. Do you have other food sensitivities?

In the Elimination Phase, we eliminated the most common problem foods but there are other foods that are inflammatory to many. In fact, it is possible to react to any food in our diet.

To test for sensitivities to other foods, you will stay on the Elimination Phase a while longer while testing some additional foods. This means going a while longer without wheat, dairy, peanuts, dried corn, sugar, fatty meats, and exceptions.[1]

The next foods to test are soy, citrus, nightshades (peppers, eggplant, tomatoes, and potatoes), and tree nuts. While you could test these foods one by one, it is easier to simply eliminate the whole group for a week. Because these foods are inherently healthy, you can add them back to your regular diet as soon as you ascertain that you are not sensitive. Unlike dairy, wheat, and corn, you do not have to keep them out of your diet until all of the testing is done.

After eliminating group II for a week, you may reintroduce and begin the testing.[2] You might test as follows:

A. Test soy.

Eat soy and soy products at all meals and snacks for two days (soy is a protein and may be eaten at breakfast). At the end of

---

[1] While this may seem trying, your body will love this extra time enjoying truly healthy foods.

[2] Eliminating a trigger food can result in remarkably positive changes. One of my students lost no weight on the Elimination Phase but lost almost five pounds in the one week she eliminated soy. Another lost 13 pounds but regained seven pounds while testing dairy, weight that melted away when he once again eliminated dairy. Sometimes, however, people simply feel much worse when they reintroduce a trigger food again.

two days, you may continue eating soy as long as you are not soy-sensitive.[3]

B. TEST NIGHTSHADES.

Eat a mixture of this food family for all meals and snacks (but do not have potatoes for breakfast and count potatoes as grain at other meals) for two days. If you are sensitive to nightshades, you are probably sensitive to an alkaloid, solanine, present in all members of the nightshade family. Do not assume that you only react to one of its members. Some contain less solanine (evoking a milder reaction) or the way they are prepared may break down some, but not all, of the solanine. This may change how strong your reaction is but, because all contain some solanine, you will react to all of them. You may continue eating nightshades if you are not sensitive to them.

C. TEST NUTS.

Eat nuts and nut butters at all meals and snacks for two days. If you do not test positive, you may continue eating tree nuts during the remainder of the test. Note: If you react to tree nuts, you can retest to determine if you are reacting to a particular nut or are sensitive to all nuts. Alternatively, if you typically only eat certain nuts (e.g., almonds), you may wish to only test a particular nut.

D. TEST CITRUS.

Eat citrus at all meals and snacks for two days. If you do not test positive, you may continue eating citrus during the remainder of the test.

If you do not feel distinctly better after a the week of eliminating this group of foods, or if you do not feel distinctly worse when you add them back, more investigation awaits. Keep a food diary and look at the foods you eat most often. Look for foods that you cannot imagine giving up. Our desire to eat a food may

---

[3] You continue to eliminate dairy, wheat, corn, and peanuts from your diet until you complete all testing because they present additional issues such as being higher in omega-6 fats or high in persistent toxins. The other foods you are testing are healthy foods so there is no need to exclude them unless you are hypersensitive to them.

reveal a sensitivity, and you might try eliminating any food you eat frequently or any food you have recently begun eating in larger amounts or on a more frequent basis. Bananas, eggs, and quinoa are examples of such foods for many. You would eliminate those foods for a week and then reintroduce them.

If nothing jumps out at you from your diary, move on to the next group of common triggers:

Group 1: Wheat, dairy, peanuts, dried corn
Group 2: Soy, nightshades, tree nuts, citrus
Group 3: Eggs, grains, legumes, shellfish
Group 4: Fish, meat, fruit

While testing foods you must remain on the Elimination Phase so you do not expand your food list (see chapter 24) until you are done with *all* food testing. Remember that any food can cause a reaction and the culprit is often a food we eat frequently or are unusually fond of.

OTHER WAYS TO DETECT SENSITIVITIES
THE PULSE TEST

If you are having trouble sorting out your food sensitivities, you might give the pulse test a try. Pulse testing is much less accurate than elimination/reintroduction testing because it only detects positive responses. It *cannot* be used to establish that you are *not* sensitive. It can, however, on occasion be a quick way to learn that you definitely are sensitive to several different foods.

First, in the morning, before eating, find a quiet place away from anything that might excite or distract you (such as the television). Take your pulse for a full minute. You can take it sitting or lying down, but use the same position throughout the test. Then eat a test food (a few bites will do), wait 5 minutes, then take your pulse again.

If your pulse increases by 10 percent or more, you are sensitive to that food. If it increases 7 to 10 percent you may be sensitive. Do an elimination/reintroduction of any food that raises your pulse.

A BLOOD TEST

Another alternative is to have a blood or saliva test for food sensitivities (as opposed to food allergies). While these tests are not completely reliable, they do pinpoint foods that are more likely to be troublesome to you. The test results can help you decide which foods you might want to eliminate and then test.

You might also look into food groupings, foods that share common characteristics. A good resource for information on this is *Food Allergies and Food Intolerance: The Complete Guide to Their Identification and Treatment.*[4] There are also many resources on the internet that explain food groups that may cause sensitivities and should be eliminated as a group. An example of such a group: Mango, pistachio, and cashews. These three foods are related to poison oak and poison ivy, and trigger reactions and rashes in some.

For the vast majority of people, adhering to the Elimination Phase and testing the first groups of common trigger foods will be all that is needed. But some people, especially those with long-standing intestinal issues, may have many different food sensitivities. Often, during the months it takes to heal the intestinal lining, these individuals will do better if they never eat the same foods several days running but, instead, maximize variety in their diet. The good news is that, with time and good eating habits, most sensitivities diminish and sometimes disappear altogether.

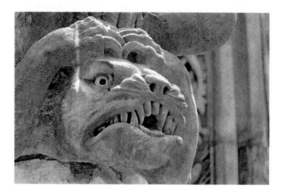

Plateau testing can be a bit of a headache
but is very much worth the effort

---

4   Brostoff J, Gamlin L. *Food Allergies and Food Intolerance: The Complete Guide to Their Identification and Treatment.* Rochester, VT: Healing Arts Press, 1999.

Does the test food causes any of the following symptoms?

Symptom	Food 1	Food 2	Food 3	Food 4
Nasal congestion				
Chest congestion				
Headaches				
Brain fog or mood changes				
Joint aches				
Muscle aches				
Pain				
Fatigue				
Poor sleep				
Circles under eyes				
Changes in body odor				
Changes in skin (e.g., acne, rashes, itching)				
Changes in bowel function or digestion				
Can you eat this food in moderation or is it a trigger food for you?				
Did your food cravings change?				
Does this feel like a nutritious food?				
Other negative changes?				

Does the test food causes any of the following symptoms?

Symptom	Food 5	Food 6	Food 7	Food 8
Nasal congestion				
Chest congestion				
Headaches				
Brain fog or mood changes				
Joint aches				
Muscle aches				
Pain				
Fatigue				
Poor sleep				
Circles under eyes				
Changes in body odor				
Changes in skin (e.g., acne, rashes, itching)				
Changes in bowel function or digestion				
Can you eat this food in moderation or is it a trigger food for you?				
Did your food cravings change?				
Does this feel like a nutritious food?				
Other negative changes?				

Part Four
A Path for Life

CHAPTER TWENTY-FOUR

A Path for Life

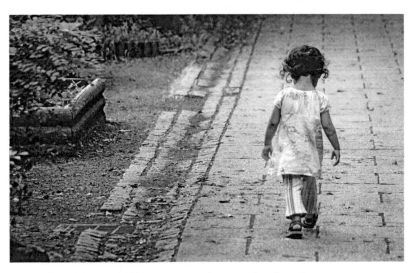

The Abascal Way, a way that works for the new you

Once we have completed the Elimination Phase and the Testing Phase (including any needed plateau testing), we may choose to expand our daily food list. We may shape a long-term plan that includes foods that are not entirely good for us. Often, if we cannot eat these foods, at least from time to time, we will abandon healthy eating altogether. Of course, this expansion is risky: It is very easy to overeat these tempting but inflammatory foods. Too many exceptions, and progress slows to a snail's pace—or is reversed—as inflammation increases.

Personally, I returned to the Elimination Phase after completing my testing because I had many issues to resolve (hypertension, excess weight, and frozen shoulders), issues that took more than five weeks to correct. In fact, I faithfully stayed on the Elimination Phase from the end of January through June. And, even today, I frequently go back on the Elimination Phase for at least three weeks at a time to make sure that I do not revert to my "old inflammatory ways," and to remind myself how much better I feel when I eat well.

EXPANDING OUR DAILY FOOD LIST

The following foods may be added to our everyday food choices:

🍎 Fruit juice, pure and unsweetened, but only in cooking. We continue to avoid drinking fruit juices in order to not overeat fruits and ingest too much fructose (see p. 136). The only exceptions are unsweetened cranberry or black currant juices, which are extremely tart. If we do not drink alcohol, we may also have 4 to 5 glasses of dark berry juice each week (see p. 268).

🍎 If we are not sensitive to wheat: Whole wheat products, oats, rye, and barley are added to the daily food list. Because they are grains, they do not return as breakfast foods except on "special occasions." It is important to review periodically the cautionary comments (see p. 242) to avoid overeating wheat.

🍎 If we are not sensitive to dairy: Dairy products are added to the daily food list. Do periodically review the cautionary comments (see p. 245) to help you avoid inflammatory amounts of dairy. Remember, all dairy counts as protein. Dairy fats should be used only occasionally to add flavor. Butter may not be used in cooking; instead, olive oil remains our primary cooking oil.

🍎 Lean cuts of beef, bison, buffalo, and venison are added as daily foods provided they are 100% grass-fed. It is important to remember that all meats, even from wild game, are high on the food chain and contain environmental toxins. Limit the amount of saturated fat in the diet by avoiding turkey and chicken cooked with the skin as much as possible. Be especially careful with any type of sausages, as they usually are made from fattier, lower quality animal parts.

🍎 Our seafood list is expanded. List One in Appendix B sets out seafood that is both low in toxins (e.g., mercury, flame retardants, and PCBs) and sustainable. List Two sets out additional seafood that is low in toxins but not sustainable. Many of our fisheries are endangered. If we do not consider sustainability in our seafood choices, many of these species will disappear in the next few decades. It is wise to periodically look at seafood websites that provide specific information on the relative toxicity and sustainability of seafood. This information changes as new information is gathered or as new fisheries are certified.[1]

🍎 We may eat one or two squares of sweetened dark chocolate (75% or darker) each day. Chocolate contains some extraordinary antioxidants and good fats that are heart-healthy. These antioxidants can offset the oxidative stress caused by the sugar in one or two squares of chocolate. (Read more about chocolate in chapter 13). Be careful with the sweeter chocolate. Many of us are unable

---

[1] For instance, the Marin Stewardship Council http://www.msc.org/ is a great resource. You can also get more information on sustainable regional seafood at http://www.montereybayaquarium.org.

to limit ourselves to one or two squares. When we eat more, the inflammatory effect of the sugar outweighs the benefits of the antioxidants in the chocolate. If sugar tempts you to eat more than you should, you will be better off eating only unsweetened chocolate, saving sweets for special occasions.

🍎 Dried fruit, sulfite-free and unsweetened, may be eaten but should be treated cautiously. For the most part, dried fruit is best used only in cooking where it can add flavor and texture to a dish. Care is needed because it is very easy to eat too much dried fruit with its concentrated sweetness and lack of fluid (water) to help satiate our sweet tooth. The result: Too much fructose. Trail mixes are especially problematic as the combination of sweet fruit and nuts invites grazing and overeating.

🍎 Non-fructose, natural sweeteners return but only for use in certain dishes. They may not be used to sweeten our daily cup of coffee or tea. Nor may they be used to sweeten tomato sauces or ketchup or soups. Added sweeteners in jams, jellies, canned corn, breads (except those used to feed the yeast, see p. 241), etc. do not return as part of our daily diet. It is important to continue to avoid added sugars in our food.

Instead, use sweeteners only to counterbalance hot spices. For instance, in Thai cooking some brown sugar is often added to balance the heat of hot peppers and the tang of fish sauce. Similarly, in Mexican mole sauce, the heat of the smoked hot peppers is wedded to the bitterness of cocoa with a little sugar for balance. Sweeteners may also be used to balance the sourness of pickles— but make sure it is used to balance the taste of the vinegar, not to overpower it and create a sweet-tasting dish. Make sure sugars are not simply added to make a tart or slightly bitter dish sweeter. Our foods should be eaten as is, not doctored with sugars.

🍎 Wine (an 8-oz glass, 3 to 4 times/week) or beer (a 12-oz glass, 3 to 4 times/week) are allowed. Make sure that any alcohol is accompanied by some antioxidant-rich foods. (See p. 229 for more information how to offset alcohol's toxicity.) If you do not drink, you may substitute 3 to 4 glasses of unsweetened, dark berry juice. These juices have antioxidants similar to those in wine.

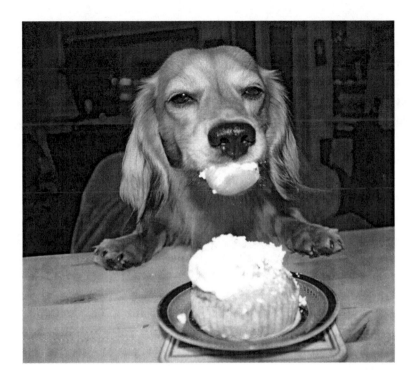

Enjoy your special occasions

🍎 Special occasions. In addition to the expansion of our daily food list, we incorporate "special occasions." Once or twice a month, we may eat anything we wish. We may have refined grain waffles with maple syrup for breakfast. Even if we are dairy and/or wheat sensitive, we may still have a cappuccino and a croissant. We may have a quiche with a white flour crust, filled with whipped cream, cheese, and ham of dubious quality for lunch. We may have high-mercury tuna and a sugary dessert for dinner. We may choose to have three martinis and we may drink them right before bed.

No doubt, we will feel terrible the next day but, if we eat properly the other 28 or 29 days of the month, our bodies will be able to cope with inflammation we generate on these "special occasions."

Be very careful, though. We often play games with ourselves and try to stretch the rules that govern how we eat. It is ever so easy to go out with friends one Friday night and have a rich dinner with a bit too much wine. Then, we wake on Sunday morning, longing for a fancy brunch. We rationalize having waffles with maple syrup because we could have had them on Friday. We decide that the cal-orie load, and hence the effect, will be the same. Then Tuesday rolls around. Our co-workers are going out for a few beers and some fish and chips. We indulge. Soon, we are making small exceptions every few days. We cannot cope with the inflammation of these regular "exceptions," we thicken around the waist, our joints begin to ache, and inflammation returns.

If you find that you are slipping and are actually living on a modified version of the plan, the best solution is to go back on the Elimination Phase for three weeks. This will quickly get you back in balance. It will also remind you how wonderful eating properly makes you feel, and motivate you to follow the plan more exactly.

Finally, try to make your special occasions joyous events. Use them to celebrate people you enjoy and places you like. If you are attending a stressful event or if you are in a lousy mood, try especially hard to avoid inflammatory foods and alcohol—"bad" foods are much more inflammatory when we are stressed (see p. 163). If you cannot resist inflammatory foods when you are under stress, make sure that you eat extra amounts of antioxidant-rich foods to offset somewhat the effect inflammatory foods will have on you when you are stressed. Also make every effort to have some antioxidant-rich foods with any inflammatory foods you eat: In other words, maintain the Rule of Proportions with particular care if you are eating inflammatory foods.

MAINTAIN PROPORTIONS

The most important aspect of the TQI Diet is the Rule of Proportions. This very simple tool, if applied meticulously, will keep inflammation quieted—often even when we are less than "perfect" in terms of eating choices.

Typically, with time, inflammatory foods begin reappearing in our diet—especially when we are tired and stressed. The protein portion of our plate tends to contain more fatty animal products of poor quality. The grain portion of our plate increasingly tends to include white rice, white bread, and other refined grains. We begin indulging in desserts and a bit too much alcohol. We grab a cookie as an afternoon snack. If we always maintain proportions, we ensure that our meals and snacks always contain enough antioxidants to offset some of the oxidative stress our other nutrient-poor choices generate. The Rule of Proportions ensures that we always get phytoestrogens to help counterbalance xenoestrogens and other toxins in our animal products. Green plants provide omega-3 fats, antioxidants, and other nutrients. The proportions help us avoid excessive amounts of omega-6 fats and animal proteins. The fruits and vegetables provide fiber and complex sugars that keep our beneficial flora dominant even when the meal contains other foods that feed the wrong strains.

The importance of the Rule of Proportions for our long-term health cannot be emphasized enough. Do not be misled by the rule's seeming simplicity: The Rule of Proportions is actually a sophisticated tool of critical importance.

Applying the Rule of Proportions requires that we always order extra fruits and vegetables when eating out because restaurants simply do not serve enough vegetables. Learn to ask the server what vegetables come with the entrees they offer. Then order a side or two of those vegetables sautéed in olive oil to balance your meal.[2] If possible, call ahead to the restaurant and ask for their help in advance. Most restaurants are more than happy to accommodate and you will not have to draw attention to yourself by asking a long series of questions about the menu at the dinner table.

When eating at other people's homes, bring a vegetable dish or salad. This ensures that you will be able to eat proportionately even if your host is not. It also helps you be able to eat healthfully without seeming to criticize your host's eating habits or making a fuss. This will help make eating away from home a more pleasant meal for all.

---

[2] Restaurants have been helping people on low-fat diets for decades now and are very used to cooking without butter and cheese when requested.

ALWAYS EAT THE ABASCAL WAY:

🍎 Eat many and varied fruits, vegetables, legumes, and nuts to optimize the phytonutrients, fiber, and good fats in your diet.

🍎 Always maintain proportions: Two-thirds of lunch, dinner, and our two snacks should be rich in antioxidants and fiber (fruits and vegetables).

🍎 There is no portion control but be careful when going back for seconds. If you take seconds, make sure that the plate is proportional.

🍎 Try to eat something every three to four hours during the day, but do not graze between meals and snacks. Avoid all foods including berries, doctored drinks, mints, gum, and food samples between meals.

🍎 Do not eat two to three hours before bed.

🍎 Continue eating high-quality protein, fruits, and vegetables for breakfast. Do not eat grains and sweets for breakfast.

🍎 Do not drink your food.

🍎 Begin to incorporate increasing amounts of exercise in your life.

🍎 Avoid insecticides, herbicides, and other toxins.

🍎 Avoid processed food, ideally even "good" processed food.

🍎 Avoid added sugars and canola oil in your food.

🍎 Save inflammatory foods for your "special occasions."

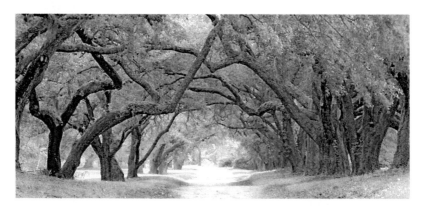

PART FIVE
Appendices

Food Fads and Fad Diets

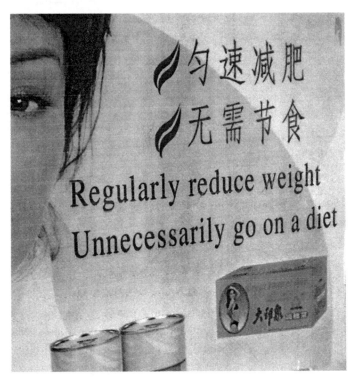

From time to time, you will be offered plans
that promise quick and easy ways to lose weight

From time to time, we are going to encounter "miracle" foods and new fad diets. They will claim to be healthy and anti-inflammatory but allow juices, smoothies, and sweet snacks as part of their diet. These plans will be tempting but only if we do not scrutinize their claims. Will they really help quiet inflammation or will they simply help us join the ranks of the normal-weight obese (see chapter 1)? Are these miracle foods and amazing diets nutritionally sound?

Begin by asking some important questions:

1. Is this a food that our ancestors ate in a time before agriculture?

2. Is the only objective weight loss? Does the plan/product provide everything we need for health?

3. If weight loss is promised, is the approach ultimately based on cutting calories dramatically?

Our bodies still thrive on our ancestral foods because our digestive tracts and biochemistry have not changed markedly since we were hunter/gatherers. They have not changed at all since the explosion of "edible chemicals." Our bodies still expect to be fed our historical diet and work optimally when we follow that diet to the greatest extent possible.

Next, look carefully at the ingredients in the products that are being offered. Are you being asked to eat refined grains, added sugars, chemicals, or non-food compounds?

Is the manufacturer proud of the ingredients in the food(s) it is selling? In other words, is it easy to find the ingredient list for the food they are promoting on the internet? Or do you only find pretty pictures of the front label but no listing of the ingredients? Might they be hoping we will give up and not look too closely?

The ingredients in nine diet products follow. A product from all but one of the most popular diet plans in the U.S. was selected at random.[1] They are rich in refined grains, added sweeteners (including artificial sweeteners), and chemicals that will inflame us—even if massive amounts of isolated antioxidants and synthetic vitamins are added to make the food sound healthy. Sugars and refined grains will put us back on the path toward insulin and leptin resistance, and will not feed our beneficial flora.

These products are not real foods. They are low in calories but are not nutritious. They are not foods our ancestors would have eaten and they do not provide everything (and in some cases anything) we need for health.

DOUBLE FUDGE CAKE:

Fudge Sauce (Corn Syrup, Water, High-fructose Corn Syrup, Corn Maltodextrin, Cocoa Processed with Alkali, Modified Cornstarch, Salt, Potassium Sorbate, Vanillin), Water, Eggs, Enriched Bleached Wheat Flour (Wheat Flour, Niacin, Reduced Iron, Thiamine Mononitrate, Riboflavin, Folic Acid), Sugar, Fructose, Modified Tapioca Starch, Cocoa Powder Processed with Alkali, Emulsifier Blend (Non-Fat Dry Milk, Polyglycerol Esters, Modified Cornstarch, Guar Gum), Milk and White Chocolate Curls (Sugar, Cocoa Butter, Whole Milk Powder, Chocolate Liquor, Whey Powder, Lactose, Skim Milk Powder, Soy Lecithin, Vanilla), Potato Maltodextrin, Baking Powder (Sodium Acid Pyrophosphate, Sodium Bicarbonate, Cornstarch, Monocalcium Phosphate), Soybean Oil, Chocolate Chips (Sugar, Chocolate Liquor, Dextrose, Cocoa Butter, Soy Lecithin, Vanilla Extract), Butter Flavor (Whey Solids, Modified Butter Oil and Dehydrated Butter, Corn Syrup Solids, Salt, Guar Gum, Annatto and Turmeric [Color]), Emulsifier (Mono- And Diglycerides [Soybean And/Or Cottonseed Oil; Contains BHT, Citric Acid]), Salt, Vanilla Flavor (Water, Ethyl Alcohol, Molasses, Sugar, Propylene Glycol, Natural Flavor, Caramel Color), Glucono-Delta-Lactone, Sodium Bicarbonate. Contains Eggs, Milk, Soybeans, Wheat.

---

[1] This one diet only provides ingredient lists to individuals willing to visit one of their diet centers. Brand names have been omitted from all products.

APPLE STRUDEL BAR:

Rolled Oats, Soy Protein Nuggets (Soy Protein Isolate), Apple, White Chocolate Coating (Sugar, Fractionated Palm Kernel Oil, Nonfat Milk Powder, Whey Powder, Soy Lecithin (as an emulsifier) and Artificial Flavor), Maltitol, Syrup, Brown Rice Syrup, Corn Syrup, Brown Sugar, High Oleic Sunflower Oil, Natural Flavor, Cinnamon, Sea Salt.

LOW CARBOHYDRATE BAR:

Glycerin, Soy Nuggets (Soy Protein Isolate, Oat Fiber), Polydextrose, Vegetable Oil Blend (Palm, Palm Kernel, and Soybean Oil), Gum Arabic, Whey Protein Isolate, Olive Oil, Roasted Almonds, Toasted Oats (Rolled Oats, Polydextrose, Sunflower Oil), Milk Protein Isolate, Coffee Beans, Cocoa Powder (processed with alkali), Natural and Artificial Flavors, Maltodextrin, Calcium Carbonate, Sodium Caseinate, Salt, Soy Lecithin, Caramel Color, Mono and Diglycerides, Dipotassium Phosphate, Sucralose, Acesulfame Potassium.

BLUEBERRY PROTEIN DRINK:

Whey Protein Isolate, Isomalto-Oligosaccharide (Prebiotic Fiber), Citric Acid, Calcium Lactate, Calcium Gluconate, Sunflower Oil, Buttermilk, Natural Flavoring, Artificial Berry Flavoring, L-Leucine, Blueberry Dried Fruit Concentrate, Lecithin, Maltodextrin, Modified Food Starch, Dextrose, Ascorbic Acid, Sucralose, Acesulfame Potassium, Artificial Blueberry Flavoring, Pantothenic Acid, Pyridoxine Hydrochloride (Vitamin B6), Riboflavin, Thiamin, Tri-Calcium Phosphate, Red #40, Blue #2, Triacetin.

MEAL REPLACEMENT BAR:

Soy Protein Crisps (Soy Protein Isolate, Tapioca Starch, Salt), Maltitol Syrup, Peanut Butter (Roasted Ground Peanuts), Inulin (for Fiber), Fractionated Palm Kernel Oil, Glycerin, Maltitol, Oligofructose (for Fiber), Contains less than 2% of Natural and Artificial Flavor, Milk Protein Isolate, Nonfat Milk, Milk Protein Concentrate, Chocolate, Cocoa, Cocoa Processed with Alkali, Peanut Oil, Soy Lecithin,

Butter (Cream, Salt), Heavy Cream, Salt, Monoglycerides, Carrageenan, Caramel Color, Sucralose. Vitamins and Minerals: Beta Carotene, Ascorbic Acid (Vitamin C), Calcium Phosphate, Ferric Orthophosphate (Iron), Vitamin E Acetate, Phytonadione (Vitamin K1), Thiamin Mononitrate (Vitamin B1), Riboflavin (Vitamin B2), Niacinamide, Vitamin B6, Folic Acid, Vitamin B12, Biotin, Calcium Pantothenate, Potassium Iodide, Magnesium Oxide, Zinc Oxide, Sodium Selenite, Copper Gluconate, Manganese Sulfate, Chromium Chloride, Sodium Molybdate.

Cinnamon Buns (recommended breakfast food):

Wheat Flour, Water, Protein Blend (Wheat Protein Isolate, Milk Protein Isolate), Butter, Yeast, Sugar, Salt, Vinegar, Cinnamon, Calcium Propionate, Potassium Sorbate, Natural Flavor, Sucralose.

Strawberry Creme Smoothie:

Calcium Caseinate (from Milk), Fructose, Whey Protein Isolate, Strawberry Powder, Corn Syrup Solids, Nonfat Yogurt Powder, Sunflower Oil, Natural and Artificial Flavors, Sugar, Nonfat Milk, Malic Acid, Maltodextrin, Salt, Disodium Phosphate, Magnesium Phosphate, Modified Food Starch, Xanthan Gum, Potassium Citrate, Disodium Phosphate, Magnesium Oxide, Pineapple Juice Solids, Carrageenan, Sodium Caseinate, Soy Lecithin, Sucralose, Propylene Glycol, Dextrose, Vitamin C, Oligofructose, Lactic Acid, Acesulfame-K, Ferric Orthophosphate, Tocopherol (to protect flavor), Zinc Sulfate, Dehydrated Strawberry Juice Concentrate, Vitamin E (Alpha Tocopherol Acetate), Cellulose Gum, Guar Gum, Sprouted Mung Bean Extract, Niacinamide, Copper Gluconate, D-Calcium Pantothenate, Chromium Amino Acid Chelate, Polysorbate 60, Selenium Amino Acid Chelate, Manganese Sulfate, Vitamin A Palmitate, Pyridoxine Hydrochloride, Molybdenum Amino Acid Chelate, Citric Acid, Red #40, Riboflavin, Thiamin Mononitrate, Folic Acid, Biotin, Potassium Iodide, Vitamin K, Magnesium Carbonate, Vitamin D3, Vitamin B12.

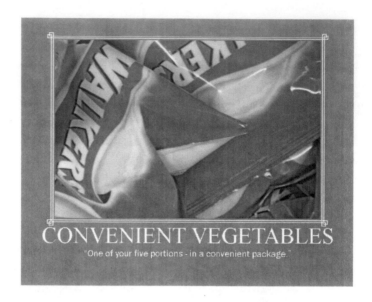

CONVENIENT VEGETABLES
"One of your five portions - in a convenient package."

CHOCOLATE SMOOTHIE:

Soy Protein Isolate, Fructose, Milk Protein Isolate, Cocoa (processed with alkali), Oat Fiber, Sweet Dairy Whey, Guar Gum, Calcium Phosphate, Potassium Chloride, Maltodextrin, Salt, Microcrystalline Cellulose, Natural & Artificial Flavors, Acesulfame Potassium (non-nutritive sweetener), Magnesium Oxide, dl-Methionine, Modified Corn Starch, Soy Lecithin, Corn Syrup Solids, Ascorbic Acid, Ferric Orthophosphate, Dicalcium Phosphate, dl-Alpha Tocopheryl Acetate, Niacinamide, Zinc Oxide, Manganese Sulfate, d-Calcium Pantothenate, Copper Sulfate, Pyridoxine Hydrochloride, Vitamin A Palmitate, Riboflavin, Thiamin Mononitrate, Chromium Chloride, Sodium Molybdate, Folic Acid, Biotin, Potassium Iodide, Sodium Selenite, Vitamin K-1, Vitamin D3, Cyanocobalamin.

PROTEIN SHAKE:

Protein blend containing Hydrolyzed Whey Protein Isolate, Calcium Caseinate, Milk Protein Isolate, Potassium Caseinate, Egg Albumen, Whey Protein Concentrate, Sodium Caseinate, l-Glutamine, Taurine, l-Carnitine and Calcium AlphaKetoglutarate, Soy Isoflavones), Maltodextrin, Fructose,

Natural and Artificial Flavoring, Vitamin-Mineral blend consisting of: Dicalcium Phosphate, Magnesium Oxide, Potassium Phosphate, Choline Bitartrate, Potassium Citrate, Potassium Chloride, Vitamin E Acetate, Ascorbic Acid, Ferrous Fumarate, beta-Carotene, Boron Proteinate, Biotin, Niacinamide, Zinc Oxide, Manganese Gluconate, Vitamin A Palmitate, Calcium Pantothenate, Molybdenum Amino Acid Chelate, Copper Gluconate, Folic Acid, Vitamin D3, Copper Sulfate, Pyridoxine Hydrochloride, Thiamine Mononitrate, Riboflavin, Chromium Polynicotinate, Selenium Amino Acid Chelate, Potassium Iodide, Cyanocobalamin), Xanthan Gum, *Garcinia cambogia* Extract, Soy Lecithin, Aspartame, Salt, medium-chain Triglycerides, Bromelain, Safflower Oil, Canola Oil, Cellulose Gum, Carrageenan, Borage Oil, Mono- and Diglycerides.

SOME FOOD FADS

There are also many food fads that will come our way from time to time. Here are a few examples of new fads that looked attractive to some of my students:

EXAMPLE ONE: CHOCOLATE WITH ACAI AND BLUEBERRIES

One student brought me a promotion for an antioxidant-rich chocolate bar. The marketing pitch read:

"Dear Y: I am looking for good people who would be interested in something I am involved with that is very exciting and wanted to share with you because of your spirit and previous entrepreneurial history … You know how so many people seem to worry about health and money? Well, I help people stay healthy by eating chocolate and make money at the same time. What more can anyone ask for? :) This wonderful Belgian Chocolate made with a proprietary cold process so that it is truly healthy has made a huge difference for both me and my husband health wise. It has helped many, including cholesterol issues believe it or not. If you or anyone you know might be interested in learning more about this Chocolate, the possible health benefits and the opportunity to make $ please let me know and I would be glad to tell you more."

The ingredients in the chocolate bar were dark chocolate [unsweetened chocolate], raw cane juice crystals, cocoa, lecithin (emulsifier), acai powder, blueberry powder.

Our hunter/gatherer ancestors did not eat chocolate bars. Chocolate bars do not provide all of the nutrients we need. They do not provide fiber. We do not know how much, if any, omega-3 fats are present in blueberry powder, and the bar is not a source of high-quality protein. It is being sold based on a high ORAC score (see p 109). It does not provide a broad variety of different antioxidants.

The bar does contain cane juice and lecithin. Lecithin is usually made from genetically modified soy using solvents, but most chocolate bars on the market also contain soy lecithin.

Ultimately, this chocolate bar is similar to dark chocolate bars that you can buy almost anywhere. However, we are not told what percentage chocolate it contains while most dark chocolate bars available at the store today provide that information. Still, as long as we are not being asked to eat more than one or two squares a day, this chocolate bar looks fine. The problem lies in the marketing angle. The sales pitch strongly suggests this chocolate is all we need for health. Many people, struggling with how to incorporate dark, leafy greens and other vegetables into their lives, will happily buy this chocolate hoping to substitute chocolate for their vegetables. They will forget that, to be healthy, they need fiber, omega-3 fats, and a variety of different antioxidants. We cannot get everything we need from processed chocolate, acai powder, and blueberry powder. The bar is not the solution to health and likely will [mis] lead us back into overeating sugar.

Example Two: Healthy cookies

This company also markets some "healthy" cookies that contain:

Whole wheat flour, brown rice syrup, high-antioxidant blend (natural cocoa, acai and blueberry powders), brown sugar, glycerine, crystalline fructose, high oleic sunflower oil with tocopherol (added to preserve freshness), water, dark chocolate drops (dehydrated cane juice, unsweetened chocolate, cocoa butter, lecithin (an emulsifier) and vanilla), fiber blend (cellulose, soluble cocoa fiber, oat bran), plum juice concentrate, natural flavors, baking powder, corn starch, molasses powder (molasses, wheat starch, lecithin), lecithin, xanthan gum, monoglycerides with ascorbic and citric acids (antioxidants, Saigon cinnamon, ground nutmeg).

Of course, our exemplary ancestors did not eat cookies. And these cookies do not come close to providing the nutrients we need to be healthy. They have fiber but we do not know how much. Again, we do not know how much, if any, omega-3 fats are present in blueberry powder. It is unlikely that these cookies will satisfy our protein, calcium, and magnesium needs.

We do know that the cookies contain refined grains and lots of sugar. They are made from refined wheat starch, brown rice syrup, brown sugar, glycerine, crystalline fructose, dehydrated cane juice, plum juice concentrate, and molasses. There are also some artificial ingredients such as natural flavors and monoglycerides.

Here, we are offered a product very high in a variety of sweeteners, wheat, and processed ingredients. The cookies also contain sunflower oil, a high omega-6 oil. Our ancestors did not eat any of the ingredients in these cookies. The cookies are not a whole food and will not support our health. My guess is that the manufacturer hopes that, once hooked on their chocolate, we will move on to the cookies. If we do, we will end up inflamed.

Example Three: The weight-loss cleanse

We are often tempted by "cleanses" and "detoxes" that promise to return our bodies to their natural, pristine states. Unfortunately, these plans usually ignore that the most difficult toxins cannot be cleansed from the body because of their persistent nature (see chapter 8).

Weight-loss cleanses usually come in sets of expensive powders, capsules, and drinks. Many incorporate bowel cleanses that confuse the repulsiveness of excrement with the healthy beneficial flora that live in our intestines. We do not want to wash away our good bacteria in an overly zealous cleanse. We will always have trillions of microbes growing in our intestines, cleanses notwithstanding. Our choice is simply do we want beneficial microbes dominating our intestinal tract or do we want other strains? If we want beneficials, we need to feed them not flush them out of our bodies. We should not smother them in olive oil, lemon juice, and salt as is done on some popular liver flushes.

A student wrote: "Hi Kathy. I was wondering if you have heard of this cleansing program—you can do a 9-day or a 30-day cleanse. Do you know anything about it—would you recommend it? The thought of losing more inches is tempting."

This particular cleanse involved taking many interesting herbs along with a wealth of supplements. It did not include laxatives and the company paid attention to quality, using purified water in its drinks. Its dairy derivatives (whey protein and calcium caseinate) came from grass-fed animals. Nonetheless, the 9-day cleanse was a calorie-reduced diet that provided sweetened smoothies and nutrition bars instead of food. On average, a person on the cleanse would eat no more than 1,200 calories a day; on some days at most 1,000 calories.

To make the diet palatable, its products contain plenty of sugars, including fructose, as well as a great deal of dairy derivatives. Their "fat burning" shake contains: Whey protein concentrate [usually provides some MSG], calcium caseinate [provides some MSG], nonfat dry milk, sunflower oil powder, soy lecithin, fructose, natural flavors, xanthan gum, honey powder, various vitamins and enzymes.

Reducing calories below our needs may generate quick weight loss, but not healthy weight loss (see chapter 1). If you want to help your body, do not go on a cleanse. Instead, take a break from complex foods, and go on a diet of steamed vegetables, mushrooms, and berries for a day or two at a time. You will feed your flora while resetting your taste buds so that you are better able to eat mindfully and well. If you are stuck at a weight that seems wrong, work on plateau testing rather than calorie reduction (see chapter 23). It is quite likely that you are still eating a food that is triggering inflammation. You will improve dramatically when you sort out what specifically is causing you grief.

THE ABASCAL WAY IS DIFFERENT

There are no short cuts if we want to be healthy. Unless we are able to hire a chef, we have to spend time in the kitchen if we are to eat real food. There is absolutely no way around our need for fresh vegetables. Our vegetables cannot be dried to a powder and mixed with a variety of sugars, fructose, and tasty chemicals if we want to be healthy and normal-weight. No matter how happy the cow, we cannot maintain healthy intestinal flora, protect our bones, and avoid environmental toxins on a diet too rich in meat and dairy.

Fortunately, after five weeks on the plan, you will know that eating well is not that difficult. Fortunately, following the Abascal Way becomes easier and easier the longer we stay on it. You will begin to love the beautiful colors, textures, and tastes of what you eat.

If you ever find yourself tempted to veer from the plan—perhaps because it takes effort and time to eat only real food—reread the rationale behind the principles in chapter four. If that is not enough, go off the plan for a few days. Feel how your waist thickens, your sleep is disturbed, and your energy level drops. You will once again choose to eat to quiet inflammation. Very soon, just as Michael did (see Appendix D), you will no longer be doing the TQI Diet, instead you will be living the Abascal Way.

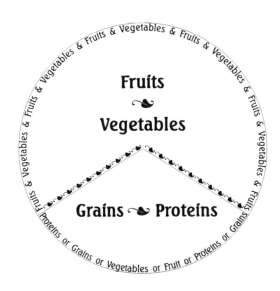

APPENDIX B
Expanded Seafood List

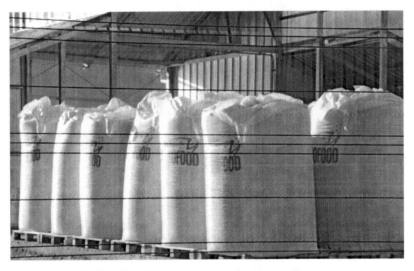

Salmofood for farmed salmon to dine on

LIST ONE: SEAFOOD, FINE TO EAT, WILD UNLESS OTHERWISE NOTED

Bass: Only if certified as sustainable
Clam: hard (farmed), littleneck (farmed), Manila (farmed)
Cod: Pacific only if certified as sustainable
Crawfish: (farmed in U.S.)
Herring: Atlantic
Mackerel: Atlantic or chub
Mahi Mahi: Unless caught with longline
Mussel: Green (N.Z. farmed), blue (farmed), Mediterranean (farmed)
Oyster: Eastern, European, Olympia, Pacific (all farmed)
Salmon: Alaskan
Sardines
Shrimp: Northern or pink
Sole: Rock
Squid: Argentine or Market
Tilapia: Wild only
Tuna: Skipjack (pole and line) or yellowfin (pole and line)
Pollock: Walleye

LIST TWO: SEAFOOD WITH ENVIRONMENTAL CONCERNS

Bass: Chilean sea (bycatch of albatrosses and petrels)
Caviar: Caspian (overfished, polluted) or wild-caught (overfished)
Cod: Atlantic (historic lows, no signs of rebuilding), Icelandic (depleted, trawled with damage to sea floor), or Pacific (seabird bycatch is a problem)
Crab: Blue (habitat degradation) or snow or tanner (overfished)
Eel: American (abundance unknown)
Halibut: Atlantic (depleted and vulnerable), Pacific (seabird bycatch in Alaska is a problem; but check, some halibut is sustainable and certified)
Lobster: Caribbean spiny (heavy pressure)
Mahimahi: (if caught with longline, bycatch of marine turtles and seabirds is a problem)
Monkfish: (declining, most caught with gill net or trawl)
Rockfish: Alaska (overfished; trawl destructive to sea floor)
Roughy: Orange (in dramatic decline)
Salmon: Pacific (monitored but well below historic levels)
Scallop: Icelandic (declining, dredges damage sea floor), sea (trawls damage habitat, bycatch of sea turtles, Atlantic cod, monkfish, etc.)
Shrimp: U.S. (trawling damage, bycatch of endangered sea turtles)
Snappers: (declining, not managed)
Sole: Atlantic (overfished), Dover (below healthy level, bottom trawling)
Squid: Longfin (bycatch of marine mammals)
Steelhead: (significant decline)

Especially avoid the following seafoods except on special occasions; they are usually high in mercury and other toxins:

Bass: Striped

Mackerel: King, Spanish, or Wahoo (U.S. Atlantic)

Swordfish

Tuna, most types

Weakfish

The Marin Stewardship Council (http://www.msc.org/) provides reliable information on sustainable seafood. You can get details on sustainable regional seafood at http://www.montereybayaquarium.org and you can order wallet-sized cards that list seafood choices on Blue Ocean's website (http://www.blueocean.org/seafood). These sites also have a wealth of information on fisheries generally. However, take their recommendations that you eat farmed fish with a grain of salt (see p. 225).

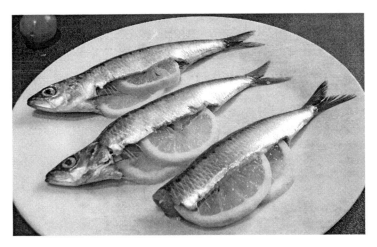

Sardines ready for the grill

APPENDIX C
Author's Story

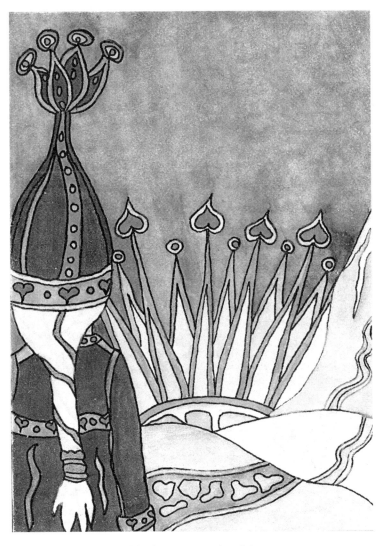

My journey to health

I began using food to quiet inflammation shortly after my 59th birthday. For the first time in my life, I had thrown out my back. My mother and siblings suffered from bad backs and had tried to describe the agony it caused. I empathized with them but only the personal experience drove home exactly what they meant. I was already suffering from frozen shoulders that I had ignored for close to a year. I could not clasp my hands over my head or behind my back. Some hugs and arm positions were painful. I woke many times during the night to readjust pillows and relieve the pressure on my shoulders. Often my arms and hands fell asleep during the night as well. Once my back was injured, it was impossible to find a comfortable sleeping position. What relieved the back pain aggravated the shoulders and vice versa. So I went to the local health clinic, looking for pain relief.

My name was called and I was ushered into the back to be weighed. I knew I had gained weight but I had no idea that I had gained that much. Then the nurse took my blood pressure. I had always prided myself on my low blood pressure but now it was 145/90. "Oh dear," I thought, "here comes the diuretic lecture." I was fortunate though. The health clinic had instituted a single-issue rule: I was there for my back, not my blood pressure, so no lecture about the need for a prescription to bring my blood pressure down. The doctor looked at my chart and asked, "Haven't you had back problems before?" He then told me that, by my age, the average American had already had at least one episode of back pain. He then prescribed high dose non-steroidal anti-inflammatory drugs (NSAIDs) because back pain is caused by inflammation around the nerves.

This was a wake-up call for me. I was getting older, my weight kept creeping up, my blood pressure was high, my ankles were stiff in the morning, my shoulders were frozen, and my back was aching. To make matters worse, these changes were basically seen as part of the normal aging process. It was going to get worse as the years wore on unless I changed my life. As an herbalist, I had long used plants to help quiet inflammation and knew how useful plants can be. In college, I studied biochemistry, the study of how nutrients work. Over the many years since college, I continued to study nutrition on my own. I had always eaten a "good" diet and I liked vegetables, but my diet was far from perfect. Now, I was finally motivated to eat to quiet inflammation, an approach that can reduce blood pressure, joint aches, and weight all in one. I would now take charge of my health and follow the adage "let your food be your medicine."

The first three or four days were challenging. I am addicted to sugar and used wine to relax at the day's end. I usually ate most of my food late in the evening and I always had a bedtime snack. My typical breakfast was coffee with steamed milk and sugar, whole wheat toast, homemade quince jam, and butter. The only part of my old breakfast that remained was my cup of coffee, now black. The rest of my breakfast changed. Fortunately, the payoff was quick and remarkable. My waist, which had swollen above the 36-inch mark (the inflammatory danger zone for women), began shrinking, and by the end of the first week my ankles were not stiff in the morning. They felt normal. After those first days, my sugar cravings disappeared. Fruit tasted so sweet that it satisfied my sweet cravings. I could eat nuts, avocados, and cashew butter (and I did). I still paced the floor at night, longing for my bedtime snack, but the eating plan was pretty easy and was working well.

Previously, I achieved my weight goal as a Weight Watcher, twice. I had lost weight before. In recent years, though, that plan had not worked for me. Progress was slow, I resented the weekly fees, and could not discipline myself to write down foods, count points, and watch portions. I loved that my TQI Diet was simple: A list of do-not-eat foods, a simple rule of proportions, and a few rules about when to eat and not to eat. It was easy. It felt right. It was working. I was jazzed.

I tend to become wildly enthusiastic about new ideas and ventures. Sometimes my enthusiasm lasts, sometimes it wears off. This time, it lasted. I continued to lose weight and my sense of well-being increased. A few months down the road, my weight loss was significant. My waist was well below the danger zone. My shoulders felt better, although I did not yet have full range of motion. I was sleeping well—I was not waking up in the night. By the six-month mark, I was 30 pounds lighter and had lost 8 inches off my waist. My blood pressure was back to low normal. My shoulders felt great.

I then began teaching the TQI Diet on Vashon Island where I live. The successes of my students spurred me on, and the program improved in response to student questions. I stayed on the first phase of the plan well into summer before venturing into the world of exceptions. I am not very good at special occasions because they tend to pull me back into my old ways. But some aspects of my eating preferences had changed significantly. I remember walking around the supermarket at the end of a particularly stressful day. I was intent on getting something "bad," something unhealthy. I looked at the ice creams. I walked down the cookie aisle. I looked at the pies and pastries. I ended up choosing a small baguette of french bread, some salsa, and a glass of good red wine as my exception. The french bread was essentially sugar but its effect was countered by a jar of good, organic salsa. There were many more antioxidants in the salsa than the cheese-laden pizza and pint of ice cream I would have chosen (and eaten) a while back.

Occasionally, I would stray off the basic plan. I would drink too much wine; I would eat too much chocolate; I would eat my cashews without fruit. My sleep would be disrupted and I would not feel as well. The minute I got back on the plan, I felt better. Then, over Christmas, after nearly a year on the plan, my sugar addiction got the upper hand. At first, it had little effect. I felt fine and did not gain weight even though I was making many exceptions each week. Then things began to shift, but I was not able to back away from the holiday foods. I was sleeping poorly. By New Year's Day, my shoulders were aching once again. Although I only gained one pound of weight, my pants felt snug around my waist. Back on the

Elimination Phase, I quickly recovered. That Christmas provided a fabulous learning experience: My shoulders' health depends on my diet. My frozen shoulders are not "cured." Instead, I have to choose whether I want frozen shoulders or health. Health is not a state that once achieved can be forgotten or taken for granted. Now, after years on the TQI Diet, it is easy to eat well. I have come to prefer the "right foods."

In my classes, those who jump in wholeheartedly enjoy the most success. They go home and clean out their refrigerators and cupboards; they get rid of the do-not-eat foods. Then they turn around and fill their homes with the recommended foods. Basically, they commit to giving the five-week plan their all. Five weeks is not a long time, and the TQI Diet only requires you to turn down foods at special events for this short time. It is designed to make you feel better very quickly and to quickly teach you how to make good, wise food choices for the long term.

The people who are most successful do not make the mistake of thinking that the TQI Diet is just like some other diet because both eliminate dairy, wheat, and sugar. They do not make the mistake of doing "most of it." They embrace the whole package.

Finally, during the Elimination Phase, I recommend the mantra "It is only three weeks. I can do anything for three weeks." At parties and events, realize that other people generally do not care what you eat. Remember, our lives are filled to the brim with events offering wine, cheese, butter, baked goods, and desserts. While you may miss a few during the Elimination Phase, there will soon be more opportunities to overindulge should you so wish.

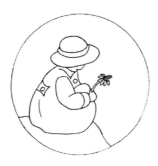

Great Results

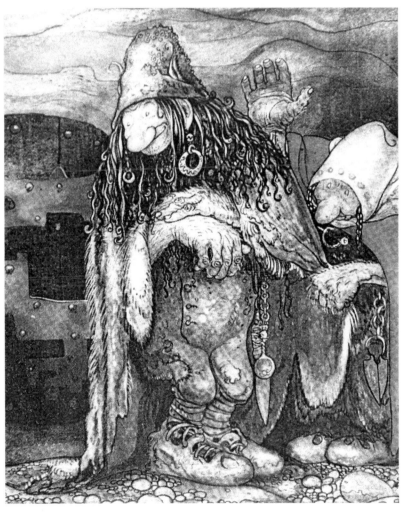

Real stories, not fairy tales

The experiences my students have on the Abascal Way are far more fascinating and inspirational than my own. I have included a few of them to motivate you.

In February of 2010, I was a Type 2 Diabetic with an A1c between 8 and 9. I weighed between 298 and 300 pounds and had for about five years. My triglyceride readings were well into dangerous levels. I had suffered from Frozen Shoulder—in both shoulders—for about three years, which physical therapy had not changed. I was taking three kinds of insulin. I took 60 Units of long-acting insulin overnight, 50 Units of long-acting in the morning, and over 15 Units of fast-acting during the day and early evening depending upon what I ate—I was only counting carbs.

I knew that Type 2 Diabetes "could" be cured with diet and exercise but I was convinced I had a reasonably "good" diet and my exercise was constrained by my dependence on oxygen—the result of childhood damage to my lungs and aggravated by years of smoking and time as a drywall contractor. I could not walk very far, even at a slow pace, without getting out of breath.

For a variety of reasons, I resolved to lose weight and, by eating less—but basically the same food—and I did manage to lose nearly 20 pounds over then next two months and reduced my A1c to between 7 and 8.

Then, in May, my wife had the chance to attend Kathy's class. Honestly, my first reaction was "Oh crap, not another diet." We had been vegetarians for over a year at one point and even mostly macrobiotic for a time and, as I have said, I thought my diet was fairly good. Very reluctantly, I began to participate in the Elimination Phase of the Abascal Way.

Within a week, I could tell I was taking too much insulin, mostly overnight. I began to cut back, 5 Units at a time. Very soon after, I could tell I was also taking too much long-acting during the day, and I began to cut that back as well. By the time I reached the three-week point, the end of the Elimination Phase, I was taking NO long-acting insulin whatever and I had cut my fast-acting down to 6 or 7 Units, 3 in the morning and 3 or 4 in the evening. I also continued to lose weight but at an accelerating pace.

As of February of 2011, I have taken NO insulin whatever for about 4 months and I have weighed between 235 and 240 for an equal amount of time. My last A1c was 5.5, well into the "normal" range and my doctor called my triglycerides "the best they have ever been." Last month, I found myself reaching behind my back to adjust my belt without thinking about it, something I had been unable to do for years.

My most recent breathing test showed a 8% increase in my lung capacity, probably due to my weight loss. I decided to try to use a treadmill and found that I could immediately walk at a slow pace for over 10 minutes without getting out of breath, something that had seemed impossible just a year before. In the past two weeks, I have come to be able to walk longer and faster and, at the moment, I spend between 15 and 20 minutes a day on the treadmill and increase that to 30 minutes a couple of times a week. I am also walking faster and faster and at an increased incline, something I would consider a healthy miracle.

I feel that the Abascal Way has improved my life immeasurably in ways I never believed possible—and it did so very quickly. I was a skeptic at first but it did not take long to realize the results it had —and, my doctor will tell you that the improvements have been measurable as well because he has measured them.

REX FROM VASHON

Kathy, I've been planning to drop a line to you for the last couple of weeks. I want to tell you how much I appreciate what TQI has meant to my life.

Before attending your TQI classes I had supposed that the significant decline in my health was an inevitable harbinger of old age. There is no need to recount to you in detail the litany of joint and muscle pain, poor circulation, hypertension, skin disorders, lousy digestion, lethargy, etc., that is all too familiar to aging boomers such as I. But it seemed to be worsening so rapidly during the last year that I had approached, by year's end 2010, a state just shy of panic. After all, I had plans for the future: I'd recently graduated from law school, I intended a total career change, I wanted to work well into my 70s if not later. Yet my health was going, going, gone.

I wondered if there was any way to fight the relentless slide into infirmity that I was experiencing. Of course I had shared my growing worries with Rosemary, my wife. When she told me about your classes and the good results she'd heard about them I clutched at the chance to attend as a drowning man reaches for a life preserver. I enrolled immediately. I was extremely motivated. I attended to the classes and the TQI religiously. The results were— well, what word would not be understatement—fantastic?

Within one week of the first TQI class my digestion had quieted and I began losing weight rapidly. Within the first two weeks my various pains and circulation troubles began to subside (no more waking up with deadened arms and hands, no more chronic leg and foot cramps). At three weeks, as I've told you, I shocked my long-time general practitioner MD with my perfect unmedicated blood pressure; after all, my hypertension records went back to the 1990s. It was about that time that I began to notice an increase in not just activity levels and physical strength but restored mental acuity, quickened, clear thought. After a month, long time skin problems on my face began to clear up, including psoriasis in one eyebrow. I began to dig out older trousers and belts: the ones I been wearing at the time had become too large for comfort.

Coming home following our first class I, gulp, weighed myself: 252.8 lbs. This morning: 230.6. So, a loss of 22 lbs. in two months (from our first class) with no calorie restrictions, no calorie counting, no forced hunger, no "no fat," "low fat" anything, no increase in exercise (still trying to improve that, sigh). Skin disorders, gone (admittedly, some blotchy redness blossomed around my nose during the week I attended poorly to the TQI). Hypertension, muscle and joint pain, circulatory troubles, IBS, chronic fatigue, all gone, gone, gone. Mental acuity remains fine—critically important as I plan to start studying for the Washington State Bar exam this spring. Most recently, just this week I noticed that some balance problems that I ascribed to nerve damage left over from a 2009 spinal disorder and surgery had completely subsided. Poor balance had forced me to curtail a favorite activity: now I can look forward to safer motorcycling again as we head into spring. The future looks bright.

Kathy, I turned 60 earlier this month. Taking stock of myself following that, I told my wife that I felt as though I had returned to the health of my 40s if not 30s. Honestly, the symptoms I had long thought of as aging have all—all—retreated or are utterly absent from my life. It is as though the last 20 years or more have taken no toll on my body and mind. I don't "feel" 60 any longer. I don't even "feel" 40. I just feel well. I feel strong and I feel myself getting stronger.

Two months back, after that first class I concluded that I really ought to lose 50 pounds. It seemed impossible; I've carried most of this weight since my mid-30s. Today nearly half that extra weight is gone and nearly every trip to the scale is a joy, a small wonder to behold. There is every reason for me to imagine that the rest of it will be gone this year, along with a host of disorders and diseases that have accompanied it. I look forward to the future. What a beautiful thing, Kathy. Thank you. Thank you so very much.

My experience tells me that you are on to something important with the TQI (I hate the word "diet" and refuse to use it with TQI). I believe tens of millions of Americans need and would benefit from TQI, if only they hear of it and are willing to commit to making the change. That change would be good for them and their loved ones, and good for their communities and their country. Feel free to use any portion of this email with or without attribution as you wish if it might help others make that change.

MICHAEL FROM BURIEN

I heard about Kathy Abascal's anti-inflammatory diet from a friend. Who had heard about it from another friend, That friend had heard about her from another friend. You get the idea. Kathy Abascal's teaching around her anti inflammatory diet has gone viral! She's a guru in the Seattle area—and thanks to the testimonials from her students, she's going viral across the country!

The diet is science because Kathy was trained as a scientist. Expect no gimmicks, she isn't hawking vitamins or super secret supplements that just came in from the rainforest or outer space. Her approach is based on food as medicine. It's the single best health related experience I have ever had. And once she teaches you the science behind what you ingest, you will never be the same. It is a life affirming, experience I wish upon all people, not just for their sake, but for the sake of our planet!

Here are my outcomes after 6 months on the diet:
Weight Loss:—50 pounds—back to my high school weight.
Arthritis: No more.
Migraines: Totally gone.
Sleep Pattern: I sleep through the night!
Food: Is delicious—and has never tasted so good!

It has been a year now, and I have kept the weight off and feel great.

ELEEN FROM SEATTLE

I signed up for Kathy's class at my wife's urging. I was very reluctant and skeptical. I did not think it would in any way affect the chronic hip and foot pain I had had for five years that had not resolved even after prolonged physical therapy, orthotics, and multiple cortisone injections.

Within 3 weeks my hip and foot pain were gone and have not returned. I lost 12# during the first 3 weeks even though I intentionally stopped all exercise to see the effect of the TQI Diet alone. Now that my pain is gone, I can run again, I have lost 18#, and I am now off Lipitor. My wife has had similar results. We both have more energy and my recovery time from heavy work is much faster. I had no idea how important quieting inflammation is to good health.

CRAIG KOPET P.T. NORMANDY PARK

M arcia reported in at one of our potlucks. A year after taking the TQI Diet class, she had lost (and kept off) 50 lbs and her husband Lee 80. Lee, a type 2 diabetic of ten years, had a blood draw the same day he started class. Sixteen weeks later his A1C dropped from 9.7 down to 5.7, a remarkable result. At his appointment, his doctor told him that he had double checked the results, worried that there had been a mix-up somewhere!

Lee also experienced a significant pain relief from his frozen shoulders. Marcia's own pain progress was slower, it took six weeks before she began to see to improvement in her hip pain but she was patient and the pain resolved. Finally, both had acid reflux problems that were totally eliminated during class.

MARCIA AND LEE, TACOMA

I became interested in the TQI Diet when I saw the results and enthusiasm our friends exhibited after taking the class. When I learned more, I thought "I can do this, I eat these foods anyway." When I heard about the elimination phase, I thought "I can do anything for three weeks and that is long enough to form new habits." That thought process is probably why the Abascal way of eating has worked for me. In the first weeks I realized I felt better. After six months I had lost 45 pounds, slept better, had greater energy and a general sense of well being. While I enjoy the occasional "celebration," I have no desire to go back to my old ways. In fact after a celebration I can't wait to get back to the Abascal Way of eating.

ANONYMOUS, WASHINGTON

At the time I learned about Kathy Abascal's classes and her anti-inflammatory guidelines for nutrition I had been living with the discomfort of osteoarthritis for several years. Walking up stairs had become so painful that I assumed I would eventually need knee replacement surgery. I was significantly overweight, and had long since given up hope of changing that condition.

I understood that the TQI Diet necessitated committing to a 21 day "elimination diet," giving up many of the foods that were staples for me, but I also knew that three weeks was a short time, and I was willing to try. Two weeks into the program my knees were no longer painful and I was able to walk up stairs comfortably. I was also sleeping better, had more energy, and was experiencing an unfamiliar sense of euphoria. My weight had not changed, but my sense of well being was remarkably improved.

Kathy's lectures covered topics ranging from the cellular structure of our bodies to agribusiness. Understanding how my body processes food and how certain foods may contribute to inflammatory conditions was new to me. I learned to read labels differently: looking at ingredients instead of nutritional information. With this knowledge my grocery shopping was soon focused on fresh, natural foods. After a few months, without any conscious effort, and eating generous portions, I had gradually lost over 30 pounds; I have never regained them.

It has been nearly two years since I discovered the Abascal Way, and it is now my permanent lifestyle. With simple guidelines and the freedom to indulge in unlimited treats a couple of times a month, this "new way of eating" has been both comfortable and sustainable.

To be perfectly truthful, I will mention that this way of eating is inconsistent with popular American dietary habits. Even widely advertised "health foods" may not fall within the guidelines. It takes a while to assimilate all the information and to create one's own way of meal planning, but, for me, the benefits of increased vitality have made it well worth the effort. I cannot imagine returning to my old habits.

ANONYMOUS 2, WASHINGTON

APPENDIX E
Biography & TQI Classes

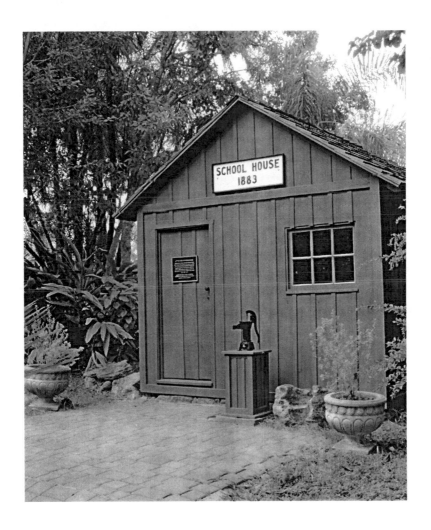

My Biography

I am a professional herbalist with a background in biochemistry, neurobiology, medical research, nutrition, and health. I am the co-author of a textbook in botanical medicine (Yarnell, Abascal, Roundtree. *Clinical Botanical Medicine, Second Edition, revised and expanded* New Rochelle, NY Mary Ann Liebert, Inc. 2009) and the author of a book on herbal remedies for pandemic influenza (Abascal, *Herbs & Influenza, How Herbs Used in the 1918 Flu Pandemic Can Be Effective Today* Vashon, WA Tigana Press 2006.) I have contributed chapters to a number of other textbooks including *The Textbook of Natural Medicine, 3rd Edition* by Joseph E Pizzorno Jr. and Michael T Murray and have for many years written regularly for professional journals such as *Alternative & Complementary Therapies.* I also write articles on herbal medicine for the general public. My passion and joy in life, dating back to 2007, is teaching people how to use the Abascal Way to quiet inflammation, to improve their health and help them lose weight. I also blog regularly on nutrition and nutritional research. (TQIDiet.wordpress.com)

TQI Classes

The Abascal Way is taught in a series of five classes, each an hour-and-a-half long. While this book has all the information you need to quiet inflammation and improve your health, taking a class can be an incredibly valuable addition to the book. Committing to a schedule ensures that you will cover all of the relevant material and will help you stay on track. Let's face it, we lead busy lives and it is so easy to plan on reading a chapter but before you know it, it is time for bed and the dinner dishes still need to be done. The reading gets put off as you finish your chores and then fall asleep reading the book.

Part of the beauty of the class is that you experience positive changes in your body while at the very same time learning what is causing the improvements. Learning on several planes (visceral, intellectual, emotional, etc.) gives you an integrated experience that has real staying power. You end up wanting to make good food choices rather than simply "knowing" that you should.

Having a set schedule of a class makes it easier to actually commit to, and do, the Elimination and Testing Phases. Seeing images during the lecture helps students focus and makes the more technical topics less intimidating. Being part of a group of individuals (a class) on the same journey can be energizing. Hearing the words helps too. Once at home, students read the material covered in class and can hear my voice ringing in their ears, placing the emphasis where it belongs. I strongly recommend that you take a class if you have the opportunity to do so.

The class schedules are posted at http://www.TQIdiet.com.

ENDORSEMENT OF TQI CLASSES

"This is the best and most practical nutrition course I have attended. I recommend Kathy Abascal's TQI Diet class to my patients, family and friends."

Ron Singler, MD, ABFP Diplomate, AAFP Fellow,
Medical Director – Highline Medical Group

Our Photographers

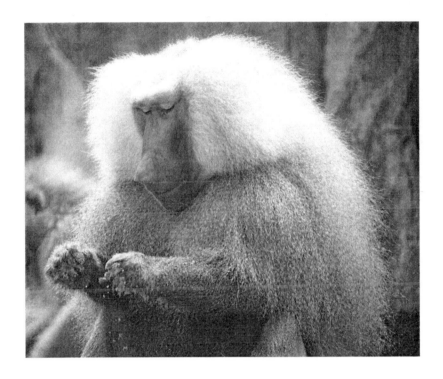

Front cover and Page 272:
A Path Through Darkness Often Leads to a Brighter Future
ⓒⓕⓞ by Brian J Buck, June 14, 2006
http://www.flickr.com/photos/bbsc30/

Page 3: *New Life – 52 WFND 6/52*
ⓒⓕ by Mark Robinson, February 11, 2011
http://www.flickr.com/photos/66176388@N00/

Page 7: *Abdominal Fat*
© by Marty Chobot/National Geographic Stock

Page 11: *Icicle*
ⓒⓕⓔ by Tehusagent, February 19, 2007
http://www.flickr.com/photos/usagent

Page 13: *Sneeze*
© by Matt Musselman
http://www.flickr.com/photos/mussels/

Page 21: *Days End*
© by Steven A. Ludewig, November 9, 2007
http://www.flickr.com/photos/sludewig/

Pages 27, 123: *Proportions diagram*
© by Kathy Abascal, 2011

Page 25: *Warning*
ⓒⓕ by Steve Jurvetson, October 28, 2004
http://www.flickr.com/photos/jurvetson/

Page 39: *The Thinker*
ⓒⓕⓞ by Keven Law, February 11, 2008
http://www.flickr.com/photos/kevenlaw/

Page 43: *But it's a healthy snack. Version 2*
© by Rick Craig, October 2, 2006
http://www.flickr.com/photos/imrickndakota/

Page 46: *A mouthful*
© by Jacky Parker, July 2, 2008
http://www.flickr.com/photos/yappingjak/

Page 48: *Jaguaress looking at me*
ⓒⓘ⊜ by Tambako the Jaguar, July 18, 2009
http://www.flickr.com/photos/tambako/

Page 50: *Madcap Coffee Raw Sugar*
ⓒⓘ by Steven Depolo, June 30, 2009
http://www.flickr.com/photos/stevendepolo/

Page 50: *Flaming Dessert*
ⓒⓘ by Rich Bowen, May 20, 2008
http://www.flickr.com/photos/rbowen/

Page 53: *Sweet! (please snatch this)*
ⓒⓘ by Gabriela Ruellan, October 17, 2010
http://www.flickr.com/photos/ultimorollo/

Page 54: *Wheat spikes (Triticum aestivum L.)*
ⓒⓘⓞ by Dag TF Endresen, July 20, 2004
http://www.flickr.com/photos/dag_endresen/

Page 58: *MY corn*
ⓒⓘ by Matt MacGillivray, August 5, 2006
http://www.flickr.com/photos/qmnonic/

Page 66: *Cooling with Juice*
ⓒⓘ by Ananta B Lamichhane, May 25, 2007
http://www.flickr.com/photos/anantablamichhane/

Page 73: *E. coli 5029*
Photo by Jancie Carr, courtesy of CDC/Biofilm Laboratory
http://www.cdc.gov

Page 77: *Apoptosis*
Courtesy of NASA
http://www.nasa.gov

Page 80: *Nopales*
© by Daniel Torres, January 5, 2008
http://www.flickr.com/photos/dantorres/

Page 85: *Broccoli Fractal*
Courtesy of Sven Geier
http://www.sgeier.net/fractals/aboutme.php

Page 91: *Robin_5654*
ⓒ ⓘ ⊜ Ⓢ by Jean-Guy Dallaire, September 19, 2007
http://www.flickr.com/photos/13101875@N00/

Page 95: *Still Life with Old Fruit*
© by Ben Roberts, August 4, 2007
http://www.flickr.com/photos/benrobertsabq/

Page 99: *Romanesco Cauliflower*
© by Harris Graber, October 16, 2006
http://www.flickr.com/photos/monkeyone/

Page 101: *50ties cigarettes offering stand*
© by Marcel More`, February 26, 2006
http://www.flickr.com/photos/marcel-more/

Page 108: *Giraffe*
ⓒ ⓘ by Marcin Wichary, July 28, 2009
http://www.flickr.com/photos/mwichary/

Page 111: *Jump!*
ⓒ ⓘ by Christopher Michel, July 17, 2009
http://www.flickr.com/photos/cmichel67/

Page 114: *Air Hostess*
Courtesy of CDC
http://www.cdc.gov

Page 116: *Two Sea lions nose-to-nose*
ⓒ ⓘ by Mike Baird, June 10, 2009
http://www.flickr.com/photos/mikebaird/

Page 117: *Oestradiol*
Public Domain by Benjah-bmm27, December 12, 2006
http://commons.wikimedia.org/wiki/File:Oestradiol-3D-balls.png

Page 118: *White Lipped Green Tree Frog*
ⓒ ① by Faye Pini, March 23, 2006
http://www.flickr.com/photos/67156567@N00/

Page 119: *Bisphenol-A*
Public Domain by Edgar181, August 19, 2009
http://commons.wikimedia.org/wiki/File:Bisphenol_A.png

Page 120: *Resveratrol*
GFDL/Public Domain by Ccroberts, August 23, 2007
http://en.wikipedia.org/wiki/File:Resveratrol3d.png

Page 129: *Dancing with Mormor in the Garden*
© by Holly Shull Vogel

Page 131: *Oranges*
ⓒ ① by Kyle McDonald, April 14, 2009
http://www.flickr.com/photos/kylemcdonald/

Page 134: *One for me and one for you*
© by Robert Grove, October, 2009
http://www.flickr.com/photos/robertgrove/

Page 141: *Mah Fridge*
© Madeline Marshall, December 26, 2007

Page 143: *Peach Drinks Milk*
ⓒ ① ◎ by Sunny Ripert, September 3, 2007
http://www.flickr.com/photos/sunfox/

Page 148: *DSC_1123*
ⓒ ① by Ben Fredericson, September 20, 2008
http://www.flickr.com/photos/xjrlokix

Page 149: *Savoy 2*
ⓒ ① by Liz West, October 21, 2005
http://www.flickr.com/photos/calliope/

Page 154: *My favorite aisle in the market*
ⓒ ① ◎ by Florian/FBoyd, July 25, 2008
http://www.flickr.com/photos/fboyd/

Page 157: *Chocolat de Bonnat 100%*
ⓒ ⓘ by EverJean, November 4, 2007
http://www.flickr.com/photos/evert-jan/

Page 159: *Making chocolate sign 1*
ⓒ ⓘ by Steven Damron, March 18, 2010
http://www.flickr.com/photos/sadsnaps/

Page 161: *Fat Boy*
ⓒ ⓘ Ⓢ by James Marvin Phelps, November 12, 2006
http://www.flickr.com/photos/mandj98/

Page 165: *Hissing cats*
ⓒ ⓘ ⊜ Ⓢ by Ingo Forstenlechner, 2006
http://www.flickr.com/photos/ingopics/

Page 167: *So... Sleepy...*
© by Kalen Soger, March 26, 2008
http://www.flickr.com/photos/k_soggie/

Page 170: *Where is she?*
ⓒ ⓘ ⊜ by Laura Askelin, November 18, 2007
http://www.flickr.com/photos/cursedthing/

Page 171: *Universal Food Chopper*
ⓒ ⓘ ⊚ by Dan Century, November 11, 2008
http://www.flickr.com/photos/dancentury/

Page 175: *Stepford wife anyone?*
© by Amara, May 9, 2007
http://www.flickr.com/photos/25152449@N06/

Page 179: *Technical Animal Fat*
ⓒ ⓘ ⊜ by Curtis Coates, August 23, 2006
http://www.flickr.com/photos/voluntaryist/

Page 182: *9aug07: giving grass with left, taking a picture with right...*
© by Guus Timpers
http://www.flickr.com/photos/oosteres/

Page 187: *Swimming Tiger*
ⓒ ⓘ ⊖ by Dmitry Krendelev, March 14, 2008
http://www.flickr.com/photos/dmkr/

Page 189: *Vet-sin*
ⓒ ⓘ ⓞ by Fotoosvanrobin, February 10, 2009
http://www.flickr.com/photos/fotoosvanrobin/

Page 195: *K7a516-6 (gene gun)*
Photo by Keith Weller, courtesy of ARS-USDA
http://www.ars.usda.gov/

Page 201: *Lemon from Chile*
ⓒ ⓘ by Andy Thrasher, October 24, 2007
http://www.flickr.com/photos/athrasher/

Page 203: *Barn owl (Tyto alba) checking me out*
© by Reginald Dlani, August 6, 2007
http://www.flickr.com/photos/reginald_dlani/

Page 206: *Sweaty Rolex Horse*
© by Joe Benavide

Page 211: *Peter Pan-ette*
ⓒ ⓘ by KitAy, January 13, 2008
http://www.flickr.com/photos/kitpfish/

Page 214: *Grazing*
ⓒ ⓘ ⓞ by Pete Markham, May 10, 2009
http://www.flickr.com/photos/pmarkham/

Page 218: *Morels*
ⓒ ⓘ by Rebecca Siegel, June 6, 2009
http://www.flickr.com/photos/grongar/

Page 226: *When you are thirsty it's too late to think about digging a well*
ⓒ ⓘ by Manoj Vasanth, October 2, 2008
http://www.flickr.com/photos/manojvasanth/

Page 233: *Honey Bee Macro*
ⓒ ① by Wildxplorer, January 29, 2010
http://www.flickr.com/photos/krayker/

Page 237: *New York. East Hampton. Pop eye*
ⓒ ① ◎ by Tomas Fáno, June 24, 2008
http://www.flickr.com/photos/tomasfano/

Page 243: *Szarotka crazy about cheese*
© by Klara Salamonska, April 21, 2007
http://www.flickr.com/photos/chmurka/

Page 246: *Aspergillus flavus*
Photo by Libero Ajello, courtesy of CDC
http://phil.cdc.gov/phil/home.asp

Page 255: *Stuck in the sand*
ⓒ ① by Alberto Alerigi, September 13, 2004
http://www.flickr.com/photos/albertoalerigi/

Page 260: Gargoyle Has a Headache
ⓒ ① ⊖ by Katie Claypoole, April 14, 2007
http://www.flickr.com/photos/clatiek/

Page 265: Walking it alone
ⓒ ① by Lance Shields, June 15, 2006
http://www.flickr.com/photos/lancesh/

Page 269: Happy birthday Yogi, he sure loves the three dog bakery
© by Dan Bennett, June 1, 2009
http://www.flickr.com/photos/soggydan/

Page 275: Unnecessarily go on a diet
ⓒ ① ◎ by Fod Tzellos, February 17, 2010
http://www.flickr.com/photos/fod/

Page 280: Convenient Food
ⓒ ① by Graham Richardson, June 1, 2007
http://www.flickr.com/photos/didbygraham/

Page 287: Salmofood – farmed salmon food
ⓒⓘ by Sam Beebe, January 22, 2009
http://www.flickr.com/photos/sbeebe/

Page 289: *Sardines ready for grill*
ⓒⓘⓢ by FotoosVanRobin, June 21, 2007
http://www.flickr.com/photos/fotoosvanrobin/

Page 291: *Northern Girl*
© by Kathy Abascal 2010

Page 295: *Anemopsis*
© by Kathy Abascal 2009

Page 297: *Trollen by John Bauer*
© by Holly Shull Vogel 2011

Page 305: *First Melbourne School House*
ⓒⓘⓢ by Richard Broderick, November 28, 2009
http://www.flickr.com/photos/richardbroderick/

Page 309: *Hello Human*
ⓒⓘ by Chi King, April 22, 2006
http://www.flickr.com/photos/davelau

Pages 29 and 30: *Clip art*
Clipart.com

Back cover: *Archway*
ⓒⓘ by IrishFireside, August 1, 2010
http://www.flickr.com/photos/Irishfireside

CPSIA information can be obtained at www.ICGtesting.com
Printed in the USA
BVOW03s1253070714

357835BV00001B/1/P